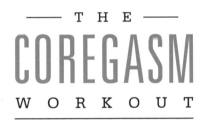

— T H E —
COREGASM
W O R K O U T

• THE REVOLUTIONARY METHOD •
FOR BETTER SEX THROUGH EXERCISE

THE

COREGASM

WORKOUT

DR. DEBBY HERBENICK

SEAL PRESS

The Coregasm Workout

Copyright © 2015 Debby Herbenick

Library of Congress Cataloging-in-Publication Data
Herbenick, Debby.
The coregasm workout : science-backed principles for more pleasurable
sex & exercise / by Debby Herbenick.
pages cm
ISBN 978-1-58005-564-2
1. Sexual exercises. 2. Orgasm. 3. Physical fitness. I. Title.
HQ31.H4734 2015
613.7--dc23
2014038926

Published by
Seal Press
A Member of the Perseus Books Group
1700 Fourth Street
Berkeley, California
Sealpress.com

Cover design by Faceout Studio, Kara Davison
Interior design by Megan Jones Design
Interior photos by Chelsea Sanders of Blueline Media
Hair by Chelsea Langley and makeup by Julie McLenachen at Royale Hair Parlor in
Bloomington, Indiana

Printed in Canada
Distributed by Publishers Group West

For Meredith, Aran, Jasmine, and Bianca:
Four very bright stars in the future of sexual health education

CONTENTS

INTRODUCTION

Your heart rate's up, your breath has quickened, and you're feeling warm and flushed. Excited, even. Blood is pumping through your body. You feel amazing, as if you could do this forever. There's a tension in your body, and you're somehow feeling both relaxed and energized at the same time. And yet this tension will soon break free to feelings of euphoria as your whole body tenses and then relaxes.

Does the above sound to you like sex? Or exercise?

There are many similarities between sex and exercise. You might even think about sex as a form of exercise. After all, sex is often fun and recreational. It's something most of us do as part of our leisure time, at least during certain years or decades of our lives. Also, having sex burns calories, gets our heart rate up, and improves flexibility.

It so happens that we can enhance our sexual desire and arousal through exercise (not just through sex), and this can make workouts more fun or motivating. Would you like to know how? Then read on.

Numerous studies have demonstrated that exercise is good for our sex lives. People who walk or jog, who swim or do yoga, tend to have better sexual function than those who don't exercise too often. How so? For one, exercising with some regularity can help you feel better about your body. Physiologically, exercise can also improve your flexibility for your favorite sex positions and improve blood flow throughout your body. (Strong blood flow is important for women's vaginal lubrication, men's erections, and arousal in general.) But our research suggests exercise has even more potential to improve our sexual lives than has previously been realized.

I work as a sexuality researcher and educator at Indiana University's School of Public Health and The Kinsey Institute. It's my job to think about sex! And as a lifetime fitness enthusiast, I often think about exercise and how it matters for our cardiovascular (heart) health, our mood, and its potential to improve our sexual lives. For the past five years, I've merged these interests by studying the fascinating and—until now—rarely discussed topic of exercise-induced orgasms and arousal. I've incorporated what I've learned from this research, and from surveys of and interviews with many women and men, into *The Coregasm Workout*.

I wrote this book to help you, the reader, learn to explore and appreciate your body and its unique and beautiful shape, size, and sensations. I want to share with you what I've learned about how fitness can help boost arousal, improve your sex life, and better connect you to the "core" of your being—literally. In learning how arousal and orgasm function in our bodies, we can create happier, more satisfied relationships and sex lives. To that end, this book also offers safe, fun exercises that both strengthen your core and just might awaken parts of your sexuality you didn't even know existed. And this applies whether you exercise often or rarely.

THE STUDY OF EXERCISE-INDUCED AROUSAL AND ORGASM

If you've never heard of exercise-induced orgasms (also called "exercise orgasms" or "coregasms," as they tend to arise from exercises that engage the core abdominal muscles), you're not alone. Although people don't often talk about exercise arousal and orgasms, the scientific research I've conducted at Indiana University indicates that far more people than one might guess have had such experiences. In our 2014 National Survey of Sexual Health and Behavior (NSSHB)—a large, nationally representative survey of 2,000 Americans' sexual experiences—we asked men and women if they had ever had an orgasm from exercise, such as running, walking, yoga, or working out at the gym. The results? A full 10 percent of women and men had experienced orgasm from exercising! Even more people have experienced arousal from exercise, or stopped just short of orgasm. The fact that exercise arousal and orgasm are not all that rare wasn't a complete surprise to me. After all, I've been researching this topic for several years. I also give talks about sex around the world—and no matter where I travel, if I mention exercise-induced arousal or orgasm someone will say, "That happens to me, too!"

Exercise orgasms and sex orgasms are both similar and different. Exercise-induced arousal and orgasm seem to arise mainly from body movements and intensity during exercise. Coregasms result from engaging certain muscle groups under certain conditions. Exercise orgasms feel physically similar to sex orgasms in the sense that both kinds of orgasms feel pleasurable and uniquely calming. Of course, emotionally exercise and sex orgasms are quite different, since sex orgasms have layers of feelings like love, lust, attraction, memories, or relationship issues associated with them.

It turns out that exercise-induced arousal and orgasm are just part of how the human body works; they're not necessarily about sex at all. The fact that physical exercise produces feelings of arousal in so many of us can provide clues to how orgasm and arousal work in the human body, and these clues can only improve our sex lives. For this reason, my colleagues and I have conducted a series of studies focused on better understanding the coregasm phenomenon. The findings described here derive from surveys conducted with more than three hundred women who experience exercise-induced arousal or orgasm, interviews with more than twenty women, a U.S. national study of two thousand women and men, email correspondence with eighty or more women and men, and studies in which we tried "teaching" women how to change the way they exercise in order to enhance their own arousal or orgasm.

Now, some might wonder what sort of people have coregasms. Are they particularly outgoing? Are they bold exhibitionists? The answer to both is no. In our experience with this research, conducted online and in person, we haven't found any common denominator among people who have exercise arousal or orgasm: they are adult women and men, from ages eighteen to their eighties; of all races/ethnicities, sexual orientations, and religions; living in Brazil, France, Germany, India, Iran, Sweden, Taiwan, and the United States, among other countries. It would seem that exercise orgasms could be experienced by anyone anywhere—including you.

Immediately after our first coregasm study was published, I started receiving emails from people who wanted to share their story of experiencing arousal and coregasm. Many said they'd searched for years for information explaining how or why they happened. These emails have continued to pour in week after week and month after month to this day. Many of the correspondents state that coregasm is a positive part of their lives, something they wish weren't so secret or taboo. Given that both the personal anecdotes and scientific data confirm that exercise arousal and orgasm are neither weird nor rare, they need not be taboo.

We've also been regularly asked whether people who have these interesting exercise experiences are in some way sexually different from people who don't. The bottom line: no—at least not from the data collected so far. The women we interviewed in our research were, in many ways, sexually similar to other women in the world who don't have orgasms from exercise. That is, some coregasmic women had also experienced orgasm in sexual situations, but some had not. Of those who had, some could climax during vaginal intercourse or oral sex; others could orgasm only from masturbating. Interestingly, some women who reported having had an exercise-induced orgasm, or "EIOs" as we call them, learned to have orgasms during sex by using their experience with exercise-induced arousal and orgasm and translating that knowledge into their sexual activities. And it makes sense: both sex and exercise involve practice and learning. If you want a good sex life, it takes time, experience, and communication. It takes practice!

Similarly, fitness is something we all have to practice or work at. And while some of us are naturally thin or strong, no one is naturally fit. In addition, the way we become fit changes with age and life circumstances.

We can think of sex like this too: in terms of what comes easily, what we work at, and what changes with the seasons of our lives. Although some women's orgasms first came to them without any effort at all, most of us have had to learn how to orgasm—especially during intercourse. (Not an easy feat for most of us!) Many, too, have needed to learn how to boost our desire or arousal as our lives evolved: after having children, after starting or ending a romantic relationship, or simply with age. And of course the way we approach our sexuality shifts throughout our lives as well. When we're very young, practicing good sexual health might mean bravely going to the gynecologist for the first time, insisting that a partner use a condom, or getting tested for sexually transmitted infections (STI). In the next life phase, sexual health might include choosing a caring sexual partner, planning our families, making peace with our changing bodies, and learning to ask for what we want in bed. Like exercise, our sexuality is a lifelong practice—something we attend to and (we hope) get better at.

FITNESS AND SEXUAL PRACTICE

So, how can we utilize fitness to improve our sexual practice? In 2010, when I first set out to study coregasm, we learned that people generally had exercise orgasms and arousal from certain kinds of exercises (very often, ab exercises) and certain ways of exercising. In the years since our study, my colleagues and I have continued trying to unravel the various mysteries surrounding exercise-induced orgasm and arousal. Our subsequent research indicates that the sweet spot seems to lie in working the core abdominal muscles and in certain features of a workout that are unlike any other.

How does that translate here? I've taken the key lessons I've learned from our studies and distilled them into the Coregasm Workout, a fun, flexible, mind-body–connecting exercise program that you can use to enhance your personal fitness as well as your sexual exploration. With its "C.O.R.E. Principles" and select exercises to guide your workout, this book has been designed for various levels of physical ability and sexual function— with the hope that, with practice, you'll feel better about both exercise and sex.

This book isn't about how to get off at the gym. Rather it's about how exercise can help us feel more closely connected to our bodies. What you do with your arousal is up to you, but learning to explore it through exercise can be helpful at many stages of life, including times when arousal and desire seem harder to come by.

Quite simply, my hope for *The Coregasm Workout* is that more people learn the truth about exercise arousal and orgasms and see these experiences as some of the many diverse ways that women and men experience their bodies and their sexual response. If you want to explore your body and its potential through exercise arousal, then I hope you'll find the tips, techniques, ideas, and encouragement here helpful to you. If you already experience arousal or orgasm from exercise and you enjoy it, then great! If you experience it and would like to control when or whether it happens, you'll find suggestions here as well. I hope, too, that some women are able to learn from their exercise experiences and find new ways to further enjoy or embrace their sexuality in all its splendor.

May you find a positive place for the Coregasm Workout in your life.

WHO IS THE COREGASM WORKOUT FOR?

- It's for those who like mysteries, enjoy sex, and don't mind getting a little sweaty.

- It's for those who want to better connect with their bodies; develop a stronger, fitter core; and explore the potential for an improved sex life.

- It's also for those who seek a little motivation to exercise. Many of the women in our research have reported that the feelings of arousal motivate them to work out more often or more strenuously than they otherwise would.

- And, finally, this book is for those who've long wondered how and why they experience exercise-induced arousal or orgasm—and whether others experience it too.

You'll find all of it here. By focusing on the kinds of exercises described in this book you can strengthen your core in the name of sexual exploration.

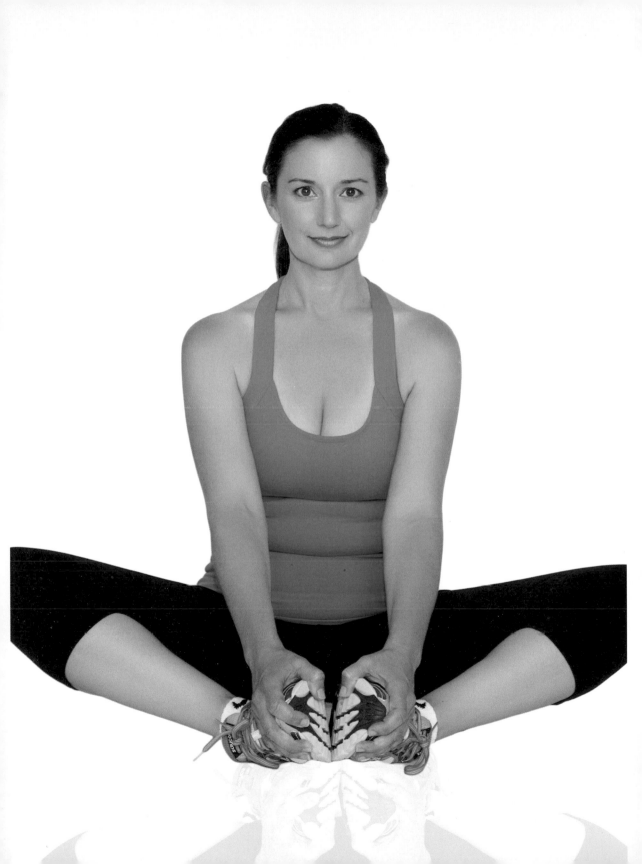

1

The one thing bugging me is I read a lot of things saying "we don't know if female ejaculation exists" or "if coregasm is real" and I am like, "Yeah, they are; I've experienced those things." It just seems there's a lot that's unknown about orgasms, something women have been experiencing for a long time.

—CANDACE

CHAPTER 1

THE CURIOUS CASE OF THE COREGASM

I N THE PAST century, several landmark research studies have challenged and transformed the way we think and talk about female orgasm. These studies have (thankfully) taken us far away from two previous notions: the idea that masturbation is unhealthy, and Sigmund Freud's suggestion that orgasms from clitoral stimulation are "immature."

In their groundbreaking 1953 book *Sexual Behavior in the Human Female*, Indiana University's Alfred Kinsey and his research team shocked Americans by revealing what was then quite scandalous data—data that prompted men to loosen their ties and women to clutch their pearls. These pioneering researchers revealed that many women masturbated, had sex before marriage, and experienced orgasms from oral sex, vaginal sex, and other kinds of sex. Dr. Kinsey also provided an early description of orgasm occurring during exercise, but he had so few reports of this fascinating phenomenon that it received only a few sentences, leaving it largely unnoticed, ignored, or forgotten by scientists for decades. Kinsey wrote:

Some boys and girls react to the point of orgasm when they climb a pole or a rope, or chin themselves on a bar or some other support. Some boys and girls find their first experience in orgasm in this way, and some of them engage in exercise with the deliberate intention of securing this sort of satisfaction. Some, on the other hand, are embarrassed and avoid climbing and other types of activities which might induce orgasm in public places, and then the gymnasium instructor may be puzzled to understand why these individuals rebel at engaging in the scheduled exercises.

—ALFRED KINSEY, *SEXUAL BEHAVIOR IN THE HUMAN FEMALE*

Instead, the quest to understand female orgasm continued with a focus on the genitals, specifically the clitoris; indeed, we could call the 1960s and 1970s the Age of the Clitoris. This was when Masters and Johnson—William H. Masters and Virginia E. Johnson—highlighted, among other things, the important role of the clitoris in female orgasm. But while the clitoris achieved notoriety, both in scientific research and in people's conversations about sex, the erotic potential of the vagina became fairly neglected or dismissed—to the chagrin of women who preferred or more readily responded to vaginal stimulation.

But that changed when, in 1982, Alice Khan Ladas, Beverly Whipple, and John Perry published their groundbreaking book, *The G Spot and Other Recent Discoveries About Human Sexuality*. This book, based on extensive research, described the erotic potential of stimulating a woman through the front wall of her vagina. *The G Spot* dramatically shifted the conversation, demonstrating to the world that, in fact, there are many ways for women to experience sexual pleasure and orgasm.

For the past few decades, these areas of research have made up nearly the entirety of the public's understanding of female orgasm: that it occurs mostly in response to stimulation of the clitoris, the vaginal canal, or the G-spot. This remains true even though scientists have looked into other pathways to orgasm. For instance, research also indicates that orgasms can be triggered by breast stimulation or through fantasy— sometimes dubbed "thinking off" in magazines or blogs—but these kinds of orgasm are mostly treated as "second best" to clitoral, vaginal, or G-spot orgasms, or even considered oddities.

COREGASM 101 WHY THE NAME "COREGASM"?

The name originates in the wake of a 2006 article in *Men's Health* magazine in which fitness expert Alwyn Cosgrove described unique experiences he'd had in the gym, and the story of a female client who had orgasms when she did hanging leg raises. After the article was published, *Men's Health* received emails from other women saying they, too, had orgasms while exercising. Dave Zinczenko, who was then the *Men's Health* editor-in-chief, has been quoted as saying, "Since the story ran, at least half a dozen women have emailed us to report that they experience orgasm during the exercise . . . It's a core exercise, so we're calling the result 'coregasm'." And that they did, in a March 2007 online article written by Adam Campbell. News of the coregasm quickly spread from *Men's Health* to *Page Six*, and then to various websites, with headlines like A Good Reason to Work Your Core and The Simple Leg Exercise that Could Replace Your Vibrator.

And yet an increasing number of research teams, ours included, have been showing there are many different ways to experience orgasm. Genital orgasms are just the tip of the iceberg! Understanding the many pathways to orgasm is important for developing a better understanding of the complex and sometimes elusive experience of our bodies working to create pleasure. Which brings us to why I am fascinated by coregasm and imagine you will be, too. Consider the following benefits from learning more about exercise arousal and orgasm:

- Understanding how exercise-induced orgasms work may provide important clues to how orgasms work more generally (even the sexual kinds of orgasms).

- Understanding exercise arousal may help therapists, doctors, and nurses create better programs to help people enhance their arousal or orgasm, particularly when they have sexual difficulties (such as after childbirth, menopause, hysterectomy, or certain treatments for cancer).

- Gaining more insight into exercise orgasms will help us provide answers to the millions of people who experience them, and also reassure them that they are not weird or alone in their experience.

All of these seem like good reasons to me and, one hopes, to you as well. Most of us hopefully experience sexual difficulties from time to time, or our partners do—which can affect us too. The more we can learn how our bodies work in terms of arousal and orgasm, the more we can take advantage of this knowledge to create happier, more satisfying relationships and sex lives.

Read on to discover answers to some of the big questions you probably have about this fascinating phenomenon and how they might relate to you.

DO COREGASMS FEEL LIKE SEXUAL ORGASMS?

In one of our interview studies, I asked women who had had experiences with both coregasms and sex orgasms—whether from masturbation or partnered sex—how their exercise orgasms felt in comparison. *Were their exercise orgasms stronger or weaker than other orgasms they experienced? More or less pleasurable? More like orgasms from clitoral or vaginal stimulation?* And so on.

One description of what an exercise orgasm feels like came from a young woman who described her exercise arousal and orgasm as "really smooth, not really strong. . . . It's not like a kicking and hitting kind of feeling. . . . It's really smooth and pleasant." In contrast, she said that her orgasms from masturbation felt quite different—"really strong, hot, sweaty, and they make me feel comfy and satisfied."

Candace described her exercise orgasms as feeling "very internal, like there is no real external stimulation, I feel it from the inside. It starts in the lower abdomen, I would say. And then it is kind of a weightless tingly feeling in my legs and then like if I concentrate really hard, it almost feels like the vaginal walls are contracting."

She was quick to point out that her exercise orgasms weren't "sexual." Rather, she said they were a pleasant internal feeling, almost like the tingly pleasant sensations you get from a massage, and yet it was very clearly an orgasm. At the time I was conducting these interviews, I didn't fully understand these tingling sensations several women described. Though I'd often experienced exercise arousal since my early teens, I'd not yet experienced orgasm while exercising. Then one day, about four years into our research, an orgasm surprised me while I was working out (and without my meaning to make it happen). I felt tingly sensations in my lower abs and then throughout my core abdominal muscles, then finally in the genital area. It was clearly an orgasm-like feeling, but it didn't feel sexual to me in any way. It felt more like an internal body massage or tingle in the way that a back massage feels lovely and sensual but doesn't feel sexual—at least to me.

Jane made a particularly good observation about how, and possibly why, her exercise arousal feelings differ from intercourse arousal and orgasms. Jane said her exercise arousal felt closest to her vaginal intercourse arousal, just less intense. When I asked her why she thought that was, she said that her arousal from both exercise and intercourse felt "more dull." She said, compared to masturbation, "the muscles are more tired, I think, in a good way. Except when I have sex I think I squeeze those muscles more because there's something to squeeze and . . . I think that's what I'm doing when I'm exercising, so it feels similar to that." She described the intense arousal she feels at times while hiking as pleasurable. "It's just not as intense," she told us. "It's like the lead-up to an orgasm when you're having sex. That's what it feels like."

That nearly everyone had a similar story of exercise arousal resembling vaginal stimulation suggests the experience is related to the internal workings of the body—like muscular and nerve activity, for example—rather than, say, to external stimulation of the clitoris.

One of the more descriptive comparisons we've received came from a woman who tends to experience arousal from squeezing her thighs and tightening her core muscles (specifically her abs and back). She wrote that the type of overall pleasure she gets from exercise—"adrenaline, endorphins, loss of control, overwhelming physical concentration and joy"—are very similar to what she feels during sex or masturbation:

> I have occasionally masturbated while thinking of the physical feeling of riding a downhill mountain bike—the fast turns and jumps into the air and reaction to the trail beneath me are similar for me somehow to the physical interaction one has with a partner during sex. It's like an incredible physical conversation where you move and react without thinking or talking. Also, I believe there is a similar rush of endorphins, adrenaline, dopamine, etc., involved in both.

That this woman's arousal can be induced by squeezing her thighs and tightening her core muscles leads to our next topic: Just how does all this happen, anyway?

Just as there are with sex, there can also be different stages of exercise arousal and orgasm. If you think about your most recent sexual experience, you might be able to pinpoint when you started to feel aroused and then, some time later, when you reached orgasm. Arousal often starts, or starts to intensify, during foreplay. Then arousal tends to build during very exciting sex that stimulates your body in particular ways. Very often, arousal lasts a long time before a woman comes anywhere close to having an orgasm. Other times, women have orgasms very quickly and almost unexpectedly—though the latter is more common for men.

Exercise orgasms can be like that too: sometimes they come on suddenly; other times they build up gradually.

Aparna noted that when she works her abs after an hour of cardio, her coregasm "comes on very quickly. It's not like foreplay at all. There's no warming up, and the fact that I'm sweaty and stinky is not a deterrent. It's just *wham, bam,* thank you ma'am."

Kelly's experience was quite different: "I try to bike for twenty to thirty minutes; it's usually around the eighteen minute mark when I start feeling aroused. Then if I go longer I'll orgasm."

As you become more practiced with exercising in ways that inspire your body to feel aroused, you too may notice your body's natural rhythms. Try to pay attention to how your body responds and when. You're the best expert on your own body!

HOW DO EXERCISE AROUSAL AND ORGASM HAPPEN?

Of course, in studying exercise arousal we hope to identify just how this response comes about. But since we scientists don't even fully understand exactly how women's orgasms happen during *sex*, we still have a lot to learn about how orgasms happen during *exercise*. Researchers have identified certain nerve pathways (like the vagus, hypogastric, pudendal, and pelvic nerves) and body parts (like the vagina, cervix, clitoris, and anus) that appear to be part of orgasm during sex, though the exact processes remain unclear. We do know this much: there doesn't appear to be one single "spot" or muscle that is the key to sexual orgasms; similarly, there's no one path to coregasms. Sex doesn't work that way and neither does exercise.

Our first survey about exercise orgasms gave us some clues to both triggering exercises and other salient conditions conducive to exercise arousal. We established that EIOs seemed to be about muscular movements and body processes rather than sexual fantasy. Many women indicated that their coregasms happened accidentally and weren't at all connected to sex. A full two-thirds of coregasmic women (66 percent) said they were never sexually fantasizing when they were aroused or when they orgasmed during exercise; only 6 percent said they always fantasized in connection with their coregasms. This is important because it means these women aren't just "thinking themselves off."

The physical movements inciting exercise-induced arousal (EIA) mattered so much that, time and again, women wrote very descriptive answers about the kinds of exercises that most commonly seemed to initiate their arousal or orgasm. One of our participants, a woman we'll call Ava, described how her coregasms were definitely about her body movements and not at all about sexy thoughts. She wrote:

> *Tightening my stomach muscles, especially lower stomach muscles, while lying on a flat surface was most effective for producing orgasm. Raising my legs while in this position would always bring on the orgasm. (No touching of genitals or movement of hips.) In later years the raising and lowering of hips brought on more intense orgasms. Hanging on a bar and doing leg lifts or L-hangs would always bring orgasm, unwanted or not. No erotic thoughts were ever necessary . . . just the muscle movement and tightening would precipitate orgasm.*

Many women described doing abdominal exercises such as the leg lifts described by Ava as particularly orgasm inducing. The fact that very often these were exercises requiring significant use of the core abdominal muscles reinforced "coregasm" as an appropriate term for many of the EIOs.

We also learned that orgasm tended to occur only after a significant amount of time or repetitions ("reps"). In other words, it took some work to make it happen. So if a woman had coregasms while doing sit-ups, it was far more likely to happen after many reps (50, 100, or even 300 sit-ups). One woman, Mallory, wrote: "I notice that I am turned

COREGASM 101 — EXERCISES THAT LED TO WOMEN'S FIRST EXERCISE-INDUCED ORGASM

Abs............................20%	Walking......................3%	Rocking horse............2%
Biking.........................20%	Leg lifts......................3%	Squats.........................2%
Running.....................15%	Calf raises..................2%	Swimming..................2%
Yoga...........................8%	Dancing......................2%	Step class................<2%
Climbing pole, rope....7%	Exercise class.............2%	Elliptical...................<2%
Lifting weights...........5%	Jumping on a	Floor exercises..........<2%
Horseback riding........5%	large ball.................2%	

Source: 2014 National Survey of Sexual Health and Behavior, Indiana University

on when I'm really working my abs. A few crunches won't do the trick. I have to be holding a plank for at least sixty seconds." This detail is consistent with sexual orgasms: although some women experience orgasm during the initial seconds of oral sex or intercourse, most do not. For most of us, orgasm is easier if we've had sufficient foreplay and a fair amount of stimulation during oral sex or intercourse or other kinds of sex play. It takes the body time to warm up, for both sex and exercise.

Another interesting finding was the specificity of the arousing exercises. Mary said, "It's definitely these lower ones. I could [work on] my upper abs for an hour and be exhausted and feel it the next day and I would never receive a coregasm. So it's really only when I'm doing the lower muscles."

That was a common experience. The women we spoke with were often physically active in a number of ways. They could describe a dozen exercises they regularly engage in that never trigger arousal. Most often their coregasmic experiences were limited to one exercise or to just a few exercises, frequently core abdominal exercises.

When we asked the women to indicate where they felt the sensations, they would often make a sort of V shape with their hands and then press their hands against their lower abs. Many women also indicated the muscles that connected to their pelvic floor muscles and groin area, and sometimes their hip flexors. We heard time and time again in our interviews that the feelings started in the lower abs, or just below the belly button.

One woman said: "If I engage my lower stomach muscles—the ones below my navel—I get a sharp increase in pleasure, perhaps leading to orgasm. This is particularly true if I sit in a straddle position and reach forward. Also, if I lie on my back and stretch one of my legs up, pulling it towards me, I'll probably orgasm after a minute or two."

When I interviewed women who had experience with exercise arousal or orgasm, one of two female personal trainers joined me for the interview. These trainers, with their years of experience working with clients, recognized that the women who described sensation along a V shape—diagonal lines from the sides of their lower abs toward their genital area—were likely feeling their transverse abdominis muscle (sometimes referred to as the TrA) working. Indeed, when we asked the women in our study where they felt various sensations, sometimes the women pointed to this muscle on the chart of core abdominal muscles hanging on the wall. Others felt that it was use of the oblique or other lower abdominal muscles that led to coregasm.

As you can see in the figure below, there are quite a few muscles involved in the core. These are just a few of the more than two dozen core muscles.

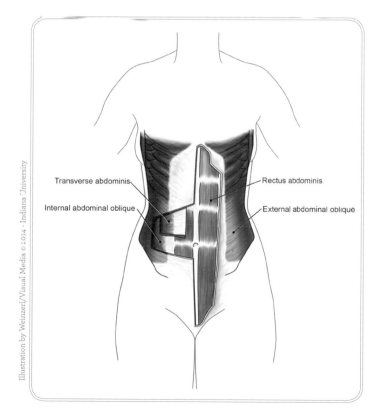

Transverse abdominis

Internal abdominal oblique

Rectus abdominis

External abdominal oblique

Illustration by Weinzerl/Visual Media © 2014 - Indiana University

Now this doesn't mean that simply engaging the TrA will trigger a coregasm. But it may mean that the TrA is highly activated in some of the more common coregasm exercises. Let's not forget, however, that coregasm is nuanced, and doesn't likely result from just one muscle doing all the work. Just as sexual orgasms are complex, exercise orgasms probably arise from a whole host of muscles, nerves, and body processes working together in a marvelous and somewhat mysterious synergy. The core of our bodies includes a number of muscles that work together in every exercise we do. Our core also supports us during sex. Again: sex and exercise have more in common than we often give them credit for.

DO MEN HAVE COREGASMS, TOO?

That men also have coregasms was startling to us. And this revelation didn't initially come from our research, but from its aftermath. A few weeks after our study—which was all about women's experiences with coregasm—was picked up by the media, one man wrote: "Since I was age four I have gotten great pleasure climbing the pole or rope. After puberty it got better yet. So, the question I have, is this also a normal male phenomenon? And if so, how common is it?"

Another man wrote from Chicago, Illinois, saying he'd first experienced EIO in late adolescence:

I read with great interest this article today on a female "coregasm" in which you were cited. I'm a male and have had this . . . for years. I have previously looked into this and was told it was probably friction—but I knew/know it is not. . . . I thought I was strange. . . . Is this unusual to occur regularly with males as well? Why does this happen? This is the first I have found of this after almost ten years of looking!

By that time I had heard from about fifty men who experienced orgasm during exercise. Most of them said they were between ages seven and twelve when their first exercise orgasm happened. Interestingly, many of the men experienced arousal from similar exercises: climbing (ropes, trees, or poles), pull-ups, chin-ups, hanging leg raises, hanging on the monkey bars, or other similar kinds of childhood play experiences. Given that women cited dozens of different exercises as inciting arousal, we found the similarity among the men's activities compelling enough to do a follow-up survey that focused entirely on men.

- Nearly 60 percent of men's coregasms happened "accidentally" often or all of the time.

- Forty percent of men who have exercise orgasms say they never or rarely involve sexual fantasy.

- Many men describe ejaculating during coregasm without ever having an erection.

- One hundred percent felt happy about having exercise orgasms, at least some of the time.

- Only 9 percent felt very self-conscious and 9 percent felt somewhat self-conscious about exercising in front of other people, even though it sometimes involves orgasm, even ejaculation. A full 50 percent of men didn't feel the least bit self-conscious about their experience.

- About 75 percent of men felt their exercise orgasms were caused by something related to their abdominal or core muscles.

In that study we surveyed several hundred men from all over the world, including Australia, Canada, France, Germany, Greece, India, Iran, Malaysia, the Netherlands, South Africa, Spain, the United Kingdom, and the United States. Of these, about 7 percent said they had experienced orgasm while exercising, another 4 percent had come quite close to orgasm, and 42 percent had felt aroused while exercising. What else did we learn?

Nearly 60 percent of men said that their coregasms happened "accidentally"—without their even trying—often or all of the time. The men largely said that they don't often (or ever) fantasize sexually when their coregasms are happening, and they aren't usually even thinking about someone or something that sexually excites them. This was similar to what women reported. And most men we surveyed or interviewed said that coregasms feel more intense than masturbation orgasms but less intense than orgasms they have during sex with a partner. One man described his coregasm response

COREGASM 101 — EXERCISES THAT LED TO MEN'S FIRST EXERCISE-INDUCED ORGASM

Sit-ups 18%	Wrestling.................... 7%	Motorcycle riding....... 2%
Lifting weights 16%	Biking......................... 7%	Squats......................... 2%
Climbing poles	Gym class................... 2%	Stretching.................. 2%
or ropes..................13%	Jumping jacks............. 2%	Swimming 2%
Running 13%	Loading an	Walking...................... 2%
Pull-ups, chin-ups 9%	eighteen-wheeler.... 2%	

Source: 2014 National Survey of Sexual Health and Behavior, Indiana University

as pretty mild: "Physically it's an increase in breath and a mild shiver for a few seconds. [It's so brief] I don't think anyone would know."

Also similar to the female response is that most men in our study believe their exercise orgasms are induced by something related to their abdominal or core muscles. As you can see, a number of women described having their first exercise orgasms when biking or when doing ab exercises, running, or yoga. For men, however, their first exercise orgasm more often occurred while doing ab work, lifting weights, climbing exercises, or running. (See sidebars for a complete list of activities likely to trigger exercise orgasm in women and in men.)

While all of the men surveyed said they felt happy about having exercise orgasms, at least some of the time, some men felt occasionally bothered by it. When this was the case, it was usually because they felt having an orgasm in the middle of exercising could get in the way of serious athletic training (for example, worrying it might happen in front of a personal trainer or coach).

Which leads us to the questions most people ask about this subject: When men experience EIO, do their orgasms involve erections or ejaculation? (Now *that's* noticeable, and much more difficult to keep secret! Women have it much easier as these things go.) As it turns out, many men describe having coregasms during which they ejaculate, even though they don't first get an erection (not usually how it happens during sex). And yet, relatively few men in our survey—only one in five—said they felt even somewhat self-conscious about exercising in front of other people, even though they've sometimes ejaculated while exercising.

Perhaps this is because, with time and experience, many men learn to control their ejaculation during exercise or else they learn to avoid exercises that bring it on. One man wrote, "I can stop the exercise before orgasm, so it's preventable in public." Another said he avoids the coregasm-triggering exercise because he just doesn't want to come on himself, regardless of anyone noticing; all he wants to do is get through his exercise routine and work his abs.

I remember one time that I was in seventh grade PE class. We were doing gymnastics. Since I was good at pull-ups (I wonder why!), the teacher had me hanging on the bar for a long time while he was explaining some gymnastic techniques. I had an orgasm in class. Fortunately, I don't think anyone noticed. Orgasm through exercise came to me years before I learned about masturbation.

—TOM

In fact, the way coregasmic men approach exercise seems strikingly similar to how they approach lasting longer during sex. For the latter, men often learn how to gauge when their "point of no return" will be. (That is, when they will ejaculate no matter what happens. This is one distinct difference between men's and women's orgasms, since women's orgasms during sex can be stopped at pretty much any time.) Once men can correctly gauge their point of no return, they can momentarily stop stimulation of their penis so as to reduce their arousal a little; by this means they can keep going and last longer. This is one reason some men briefly pause or switch positions during sex; it reduces sensation in their penis, thereby giving themselves a little break so they can last longer. This seems to be how some men approach exercise, too. For example, one man wrote of using a similar technique with exercise:

> *I avoid exhaustive exertion when I do captain's chair (but I still do them). I don't do full sit-ups in my routine anymore because of my back, but I do have to do them for the Air Force fitness test. I remember getting close to orgasm a couple times and I simply stopped so I wouldn't orgasm. I can tell when the "point of no return" is coming close, so I can stop before reaching it.*

The fact that this man notes his point of no return in exercise suggests he's pretty aware of his own bodily sensations. This is likely an asset for him as part of sex as well.

That's the power of learning about your body and your sexual response through exercise. The more closely we connect to our physical and emotional sensations, the better we become at distinguishing different levels of arousal. That self-awareness can help all of us—no matter our gender—to feel more empowered about sex and to be better partners.

ARE EXERCISE AROUSAL AND COREGASM RARE?

In my years working as a sex columnist for *Men's Health* magazine, *Time Out Chicago*, and *Kinsey Confidential*, I often heard from people who'd experienced orgasm while exercising. Their two main questions were *How does this happen*? and *Is this unusual*?

Coregasm is not rare—a realization that still surprises many people. Back in the 1950s, Alfred Kinsey and colleagues speculated that at least 5 percent of women had had orgasms during exercise. But from the sex survey my team at Indiana University conducts each year, wherein we ask thousands of Americans dozens of questions about their sex lives, we've found that about 10 percent of both women and men have experienced EIO at least once in their lives. It's likely that many more have experienced exercise-induced arousal.

WHAT EXERCISES LEAD TO EXERCISE AROUSAL AND COREGASM?

You've probably heard the saying, "Variety is the spice of life." When it comes to sex, research has shown that sexual variety—kissing, oral sex, erogenous touching, intercourse—increases potential for orgasm. Similarly, when it comes to exercise, many different activities can enhance arousal or orgasm, and different activities work for different people. Women have described all sorts of exercises that helped them feel aroused, including biking, dancing, Pilates, running, swimming, yoga, chin-ups, crunches, leg raises, pull-ups, and more. Some women even reported sexual pleasure or arousal from mopping, shoveling, raking leaves, and snowboarding!

One woman described feeling aroused from "certain full-body but core-specific actions like raking, shoveling, vacuuming. Sexual pleasure is sporadic with these activities, but present enough—maybe once out of every eight times or so."

Another woman wrote about having orgasmed while using a whisk to beat egg whites, noting it as "one of the less obvious pleasures of home baking."

A number of women and some men had coregasms while doing leg lifts or knee-ups on the Roman Chair (also called the Captain's Chair). As one woman described it:

The Roman Chair is a piece of equipment found in most gyms. It's like a pair of tall, vertical, parallel bars with little knobs sticking out. You rest your forearms on the knob parts (they stick out pretty far) and then you bring your knees up to your chest, keeping your arms stiff, and using your abdominal muscles to control your lower body. There are a couple different exercises you can do, but my way is to just bring my knees to my chest, then try to put my legs straight out—like in a pike—and then back in and back down, and just keep repeating that. That always makes me orgasm. I can, of course, stop, if I just stop doing the exercise. But if I keep going for a couple reps, maybe like ten, I'll definitely orgasm. I used to be pretty embarrassed about it but then I told some of the other girls on the rugby team and they all said they experience the same thing, although not all with the Roman Chair.
—TONYA

If you're curious to try the Captain's Chair/Roman Chair, make sure to ask a personal trainer to show you good form, as you could injure yourself using poor form.

Again, what works for one person may not always work for another. But whether it's chair pull-ups, crunches, or raking leaves, the activities do share a common denominator: they intensely work the core abdominal muscles.

Exercise orgasm happens when I intensely contract the pelvic floor whilst bilaterally contracting my leg extensors. I could do this quite easily in my late teens and twenties.
—TESSA

I usually orgasm from doing ab exercises that work out my lower abs. Backward crunches, leg lifts while lying flat on my back while engaging my abs, having my legs up while lying on the ground and lifting my butt. Plus certain kinds of sit-ups do it.
—ALYSSA

Simultaneously tensing my lower abdominal muscles and bringing both legs toward my chest would do it—but only after a certain level of exertion.
—VASHTI

Lower abdominal exercises are pleasurable in general. I'm not thinking about anything sexual, or stimulating myself in any way. It just happens with friction and muscle fatigue. I usually start feeling it during the second or third set when my muscles are beginning to strain. Vertical/standing exercises are more intense for me, but I can feel pleasure when lying down as well.
—SHANA

A regular crunch with stationary legs doesn't work for me. Leg lifts were the first exercise I ever experienced an orgasm during. I need to be engaging my core as well as my legs in some way. If I've already done some abdominal exercises, I can also orgasm from doing push-ups using a stability ball.
—MONICA

Any long, sustained work on my legs—like rollerblading or biking—will eventually start to make my vagina muscles contract. It has to be longer than forty minutes.
—CHLOE

In one instance, I was shoveling gravel from a truck into a pit, which required heavy lifting along with twisting. We were in a hurry, so I could not take breaks to rest . . . which resulted in a very marked orgasmic response. Running has consistently caused this response as well, but not as powerful as lifting and twisting. It always happens at about mile 2.5 of a light run. It feels as though the muscles are

pulling at the G-spot itself. Once I noticed this phenomenon, I started to focus on the sensation and found that I could "make" or "allow" the orgasm to happen by being open to the idea . . . and sustaining the physical action that caused it.
—KATARINA

I am turned on when I'm really working my abs. My guess is that since my abs are typically flexed during sex, I associate prolonged core workouts with pleasure. Another reason might be because I feel sexy at a gym or while I am working out by keeping my body in tip-top condition.
—MALLORY

We're all a little different—and that's a lovely thing. Different activities in different configurations. Different responses: many experience arousal; some even experience orgasm. But one thing is shared in common: once a person discovers what works, it tends to be pretty dependable—much like a particular position in sex.

WHEN DO PEOPLE FIRST EXPERIENCE EXERCISE AROUSAL AND COREGASM?

According to our research, the average age at which men recall having their first exercise-induced orgasm is sixteen. For women, the average is a bit older—about twenty-two. The full range of ages of women's first experience is from as young as nine to as old as seventy. Across our studies, we heard again and again that exercise arousal and EIOs are often first experienced in childhood or adolescence. Most of the adults I interviewed said they didn't realize until years later—when they were older and sexually experienced—what that funny feeling had been. How's that for an aha moment! They hadn't thought of the feelings as sexual because they weren't—they were just pleasurable "ticklish" feelings that happened while they were climbing poles or ropes on playgrounds, swinging on swing sets, spinning in circles, or climbing trees in their backyard. Steven shared his first memory:

I think the first experiences were at the age of eight or nine, that something "feels weirdly strange" when climbing for a long time on a rope. Definitely not because of the friction of the penis, but related to the core muscles. I was always aware of that. I actually never really felt there is such a big deal about it and considered it to be normal.

An interesting aspect of these early experiences is how young girls and boys make sense of their bodies. As children don't usually know what physical arousal is, they come up with other ways of describing their feelings and body sensations, such as what they experience when they touch their genitals out of curiosity, a normal, common, and frequent behavior among very young children. After all, sexuality doesn't come out of nowhere when we turn eighteen or fall in love. It's inside us all along, unfolding slowly as we age and develop.

But unfortunately, not all parents see masturbation or bodily exploration as normal; the American Academy of Pediatrics frequently publishes articles to reassure parents of this common behavior. When the adults in our study first experienced exercise-induced arousal or orgasm as children, they almost never told their parents because the feelings were connected to their "private parts."

For instance, a woman named Nina said she used to have orgasms when she was in eighth grade from doing dozens of sit-ups in her room at night.

I just remember I used to get very intense feelings, and my body would just stop, and I would be very tired. I didn't want to talk to my mom about it because . . . I didn't know if it was normal, and I didn't know if I was doing anything wrong at the time. I just felt like maybe it was a part of sex that I wasn't supposed to be doing, because I knew it was a feeling that I never had normally. . . . Then I got to college and I was like, "Oh wow, so that's what it was." I actually learned it in my human sexuality class. And when I had my first . . . masturbation or whatever, it made me think, "Hey, this is the same kind of feeling."

Another woman had experienced orgasms from climbing poles as a child. She specified that the climbing didn't involve rubbing her genitals against the pole, so the arousal didn't stem from that; the feelings radiated from her lower abdominal muscles. As an adult, she installed a pull-up bar in a doorway of her apartment so that she could experience coregasms anytime she wanted. For her this was particularly pleasurable because she had been unable to experience orgasm with a sexual partner—though she and her boyfriend had playfully included her coregasms in their foreplay. What a perfect example of how exercise-induced arousal isn't just for the gym: plenty of women and men find ways to make it sexy at home with their partner.

HOW DO PEOPLE FEEL ABOUT HAVING COREGASMS?

One of the primary questions in our research studies was how women felt about having orgasms or arousal while exercising. We were pleased to learn that 94 percent of the women in our study felt happy about their experience, at least some of the time. Rarely did women say they *never* felt happy about it, which could result from a number of factors.

We know that some women feel shame or guilt about any kind of sexual or genital sensations—a response often powerfully influenced by religious and cultural beliefs. Issues of sexual shame can be very complex, and are often deeply tied to a woman's particular upbringing.

For example, Aparna, who had attended a strict religious school where students were taught many negative things about sexuality, said that the first time she accidentally experienced an orgasm from exercising—during squats with hand weights—she felt "like a slut"—so much so that she dressed conservatively for the week following.

In another example, I came across a message board where a Mormon woman wrote to ask if her coregasms counted as a sin, as she had chosen to avoid both masturbation and sex before marriage. A Mormon therapist replied that she didn't think coregasms were a problem, just as they both noted that men's wet dreams weren't a problem.

On the other hand, the shame one study participant, Susan, felt about her sexuality was such that her coregasmic experiences felt like a safe haven. She said she enjoyed her swimming arousal and orgasms because they felt pleasurable and natural and free of shame, whereas she didn't feel as comfortable masturbating or having sex with her boyfriend. She said, "I would rather go exercise than just masturbate in my

At first I was just focused on the exercise and getting the exercise done. But when I figured out what was happening . . . I started doing it for the end result. . . . I feel like I'm getting two benefits. I'm exercising, getting some sort of muscles worked, plus I'm getting happiness at the end. It's the best of both worlds.

—TARA

We've spoken with several women who fantasize while running, often to keep themselves engaged, particularly during long runs. A few coregasmic women have said they use fantasy to further the beginnings of exercise-induced arousal, thinking sexy thoughts in order to push themselves into more intense arousal. Other women treat exercise and its associated arousal as a sort of foreplay, to be explored soon after when they get home. Exercise: the new foreplay!

house. . . . I don't know, it's really awkward. I don't feel comfortable masturbating in my house, even in my room. I feel like someone's going to come to my room."

Even when she locked the door she felt too uncomfortable to masturbate at home, as she worried someone might hear her or try to come in. Plus there was the weight of her mother's words, the way she was raised to focus on studying and having a successful career, and the way she was encouraged to stay away from boys and sex. All this made exercise orgasms a safe, logical, healthy, and natural form of sexual expression and release for her.

Though shame around the experience was limited to just a few people, plenty of other women and men reported they just felt "odd" about their experience, often because they didn't know if others experienced it as well or if they were unusual. Luckily, once these individuals mentioned their experience to a supportive partner or a good friend, many received positive responses of interest or even envy. Some men showed their wives their unique "gift"! And some women felt empowered when their friends asked if they could teach them how to coregasm; some were even told their friends had experienced it too, just from different exercises. And though these individuals still sometimes felt "different" from others, now it was in a good way. Almost all the women we heard from said that, once they learned others had had similar experiences, they felt greatly relieved about being "normal."

It's for such women that I am moved to share what we've learned in these research studies. My hope is for women to feel less awkward—and more proud—about their sexuality. All too often women have been made to feel ashamed about their bodies or their sexuality; that has to stop. I hope that you can learn to embrace your own personal "gifts" or "quirks" related to your body or your sexuality. The fact that so many women and men—without even trying—have this normal, natural response while exercising is a good reminder that arousal is a normal, natural part of being human.

CAN COREGASMS IMPROVE MY SEX LIFE?

There are two angles to consider regarding if and how having coregasms can improve one's sex life—beyond the simple answer yes, they can. The first angle is easy: exercise-induced arousal can make for an effective precursor to sex-induced arousal. Consider how fun anticipation can be! In the same way that foreplay can be a valuable aspect of the sexual experience, many people use their exercise-induced arousal as an appetizer to build desire for sex. For example, one woman said she enjoys using weight machines that exercise the inner and outer thighs, and then frequently wants to have sex afterward.

For the second angle, we're fortunate in how much exercise orgasms and sex orgasms inform each other. I mentioned earlier that not all women have experienced sexual orgasm, and that even those who orgasm from one approach might take a while to learn to respond with other approaches. Sexual-health professionals have a number of tips and techniques to suggest to women (and some men) who want to experience orgasm. These often concern encouraging women to masturbate with their own fingers or with a vibrator. While this can help many women learn to experience orgasm during masturbation, these strategies are less effective at helping women learn to orgasm during intercourse unless they can replicate the same technique with their partner. Plus, many women seek a "hands-free" orgasm so they can use their hands elsewhere; some, too, wish to avoid the noise of a vibrator.

Coregasms may prove to be a more effective means of teaching women how to reach sexual climax. For one thing, they're hands-free to begin with. In addition, there are many similarities between some arousal-inducing exercises and common sex positions. For example, the position for crunches starts out with lying on one's back, often with bent knees, which is quite close to being the partner on the bottom in missionary position. Similarly, the prone plank is akin to being on top in missionary position. Standing-forward bends in yoga are similar to standing sex positions. And the more gymnastic and complicated plough position of yoga, with one's legs flipped over one's head, is also

You won't need any special equipment to do the Coregasm Workout. If you'd like to use a balance trainer, medicine ball, free weights, stability ball, or gym equipment, these options will be covered. Some people like to use equipment simply because it mixes up their routine and helps keep exercise interesting. If novelty and diversity helps motivate you, or if a healthcare provider, physical therapist, or personal trainer has suggested you work on your balance through a balance trainer, then you might want to consider that. You will know what's best for you.

If you're relatively new to exercise or are worried about falling, stick to the floor. You don't need to get on a stability ball or a balance trainer to have a good workout, and keeping your feet planted on the ground can be safer. If you're trying to increase strength, that can be done more easily and effectively standing on the floor.

If you choose to use the balance trainer, know that just trying to keep your balance can be work enough; you might find it too distracting to experience arousal or orgasm. Then again, it may be just the challenge you need to get there. As Christy said, "It is very challenging for me to get an orgasm from a regular push-up, but when I do a push-up where my hands or feet are on a stability ball, it can happen. I often need to tense up my core very tightly until I am almost shaking/vibrating."

Remember: exercise arousal and orgasms are diverse and come from all sorts of exercises, so choose to explore exercises that feel safe, healthy, and enjoyable to you.

similar to a sex position that many people enjoy. Learning to experience arousal with these kinds of exercises may provide a pathway from the gym to the bedroom.

Sometimes it's not about a specific position, but the more subtle movements within the body. For example, one woman reported she has exercise orgasms by first engaging her ab and pelvic floor muscles and then stretching until she feels a strain in her thighs and hamstrings; in pushing for further strain beyond that, she can reach orgasm. Given this description, it's easy to imagine translating some of these same movements into sex by engaging one's abdominal and pelvic floor muscles, as well as the thigh muscles.

A specific aspect of this lesson application is being sensitive to how the smallest changes in movement can produce different sensations. For example, some women simply noticed a similarity between what they do in sex and what they do in exercise. One wrote:

I was riding my horse, bareback, . . . and trying out different positions to find the most comfortable for the horse's different gaits. I found that relaxing my hips, tensing my lower abdominal muscles, and leaning back slightly (one of the more common positions advised for bareback riding) led to pleasurable friction. However, I think most of the effect was because of the tenseness in my abdominal muscles. Holding these muscles rigid is something I also do during sexual activity (by myself and/or with a partner) to become aroused or orgasm.

This attention to the particular effect of minimal shifts in position is as important to our sexual development as learning what kinds of sexual behaviors we like—oral sex, sex-toy play, breast play, sex positions, etc.—as well as what kinds of touches or licks we respond to.

Of course, exercise orgasms and arousal can be pleasurable and satisfying for their own sake. Many feel arousal adds a little joy or motivation to otherwise routine exercise. For example, one woman wrote:

At a certain point while running, the motion of my thighs rubbing together, along with the feeling of tiredness/runner's high in my legs, becomes intensely sexual. I have no idea what I'm doing aside from running to somewhere near the point of exhaustion and being out of shape enough that my thighs are rubbing together. Obviously on a bicycle there is direct stimulation of my vulva and the tiredness of my legs. I have yet to climax from all this, but damn does it feel good.

Again, exercise doesn't have to be goal-oriented. It's perfectly fine to focus on and be mindful about the pleasure (as you will learn from C.O.R.E. Principle 3) and to appreciate the experience for what it is. And, if you want to try to take your arousal further and deeper, that choice is yours as well.

CAN ANYONE HAVE EXERCISE-INDUCED AROUSAL OR ORGASMS?

I believe that most women can learn to experience arousal from exercise. What's more, many can develop exercise-induced arousal within a short period of time. In one of my studies, more than 60 percent of women started experiencing exercise-induced arousal *within just a few weeks* of learning new ways of exercising. Some of these women were runners. Others were yoga enthusiasts. Quite a few preferred cardio machines and ab workouts at the gym. Of course, everyone is different—and what works for you may be different from what works for other women. That's exactly why it's important to read through the C.O.R.E. Principles in the next chapters, so you can start with a foundation of how certain ways of exercise might pay off for you. In the upcoming chapters you'll find loads of suggestions for expanding your arousal and orgasm potential, including specific exercises, how many to do, and in what order. You'll also find that the program is flexible enough to be tailored to exactly what works best for you. Whether you like ab workouts, cardio machines, swimming, jogging, yoga, Pilates, or dancing, you can learn to tap into these core sexual feelings.

Ultimately, whether or not you achieve coregasm, there are many good health reasons to include core exercises in your workout. We all want to stay healthy, reduce our risk of injury, and avoid lower back pain if at all possible. Whether or not you discover exercise-induced arousal, you can still feel sexy or empowered working out, as you're likely to develop an awareness of your body and how it moves and flows through exercise. And even that is pretty sexy!

Because of my coregasm experiences, I was able to really learn about my body—the way it works, what exercises I can get it in, how fast it will take me. And so when I started having more consistent sex I was able to work my body and kind of push myself and tense my muscles to receive a stronger or faster orgasm during sex. And it's been great because my partner and I are able to, most of the time, receive orgasm at the same time because I can purposely be like, "Oh, you're going, okay," and really tense my muscles hard and receive an orgasm. He's always like, "Well is it me or is it your coregasm?" And you know, at the end of the day it doesn't really matter. It's probably a little bit of both; it's probably tensing my muscles and [him] at the same time.

—**MARY**

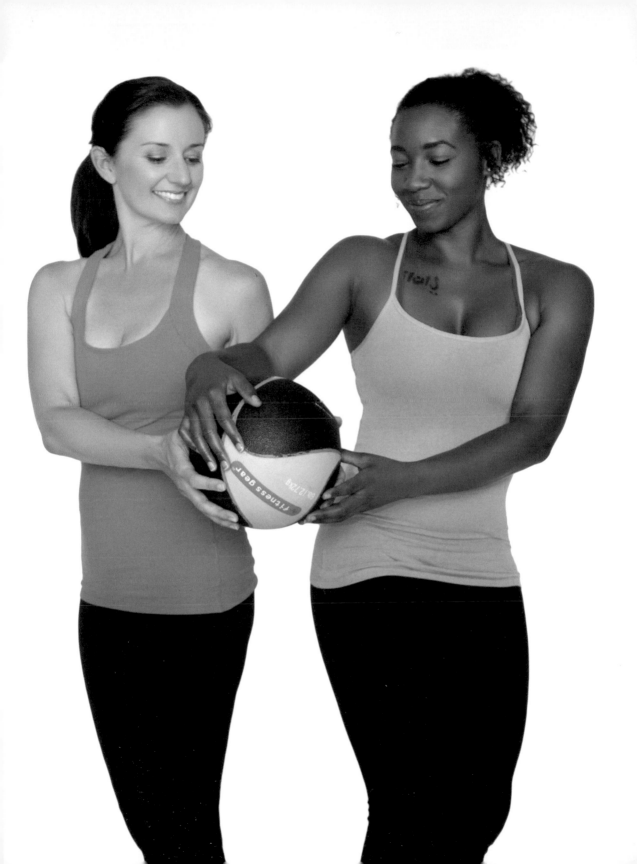

2 The first chance I had to Google more information about what had happened to me, I was stunned—amazed at your research, yet also shocked that there was not more research. . . . By becoming more in touch with ourselves, women will be able to give themselves pleasure in the most pure way. . . . I encourage you to keep researching for me, and for all women around the world who deserve to know more about their bodies and come into touch with them.

—EDEN

CHAPTER 2

INTRODUCTION TO THE
C.O.R.E. PRINCIPLES

THE RESEARCH BEHIND THE PRINCIPLES

Before we get to the fun part—when I introduce you to the Coregasm Workout, which I'll do soon enough—I'd like to share how I developed the four C.O.R.E. Principles that make up the workout program.

I mentioned earlier that some of our findings derived from interviews with more than twenty women who experience exercise-induced arousal and orgasm. During the summer of 2013, women spanning five decades of life—between the ages of eighteen and sixty-eight—visited our Coregasm Lab, where they walked us through, just for demonstration purposes and not to the point of orgasm, the exact activities that elicited their arousal. For example, take leg raises. It's one thing for a woman to write in a survey that she orgasms from doing leg raises. It's an entirely different matter to discover, during an interview and an exercise demonstration, whether she lifts her leg quickly or in a slow, controlled manner; whether she holds her breath, breathes slowly, or breathes quickly; and how she holds her posture. Ultimately, the interviews provided insight into the kinds of exercises that induced arousal, how the women did these exercises, how many reps they did, and how intensely they had to exercise to reach that point—all of which will be expanded upon here.

With me for each of the interviews was one of two female personal trainers from Indiana University's Department of Kinesiology, the study of exercise science. We'd teamed up in order to approach our subject—exactly which combinations of movements could elicit arousal—from two different angles. Between my expertise in sex and orgasm and their expertise in exercise, we were able to ask our interviewees all the right questions we needed to discover more about exercise orgasms—and, ultimately, to uncover information to help women like you with their own fitness and sexual exploration.

Later on came my coregasm diary study, for which I recruited twenty-seven women, ages eighteen to sixty, who exercised somewhat regularly and had never experienced exercise arousal/orgasm. The goal? To see if exercise arousal could be taught. My research assistants and I asked women about their current exercise routine, including what kinds of exercise they tended to do and roughly how often, and for how long, they exercised. For example, one woman said she would ride her bike to and from campus but also did yoga. Others had gym routines where they did some mix of cardio and strength training. We listened to their exercise routine and then asked them to consider modifying their exercises in certain ways.

We asked each woman to incorporate, over the course of her next ten workouts, a few modifications to her specific exercise routine. For example, if a woman normally did a cardio routine, we asked her to do it for at least thirty minutes—forty-five minutes for biking and spinning—and immediately after to do as many as possible of various abdominal exercises *to the point of muscle fatigue*. If a woman engaged in strength training, such as lifting weights, we asked her to choose a weight that was slightly demanding or difficult but not painful or uncomfortable, specifying that we wanted her to challenge herself and, again, go to the point of muscular fatigue if possible. Women who engaged in ab or core exercises also were asked to do as many as they could to the point of fatigue. In addition, we asked each woman to keep an exercise diary documenting the details of her workout, noting exactly when and how she experienced arousal or even orgasm.

The results were tremendous. Thanks to the diaries kept by these women—these pioneers in our research—we learned that making small changes in an exercise routine could produce remarkable changes in women's awareness of bodily sensations. For example:

- More than 60 percent of women who followed our program experienced exercise-induced arousal within just ten workouts.

- Of that 60 percent who experienced EIA, about two-thirds noted arousal during at least five of their ten workouts.

- Over the course of ten workouts, one of the twenty-seven women came close to exercise-induced orgasm; a second woman experienced several coregasms.

THE COREGASM WORKOUT

Now how can we apply all these findings to you and your life? In the pages to follow you'll encounter the Coregasm Workout, which I developed to be flexible and easily adapted into existing exercise routines—whether you're a yoga devotee, an avid hiker, or someone who can't get enough of the gym.

The specifics gleaned from our research informed the workout program's C.O.R.E. Principles. C.O.R.E. stands for the four essential elements conducive to eliciting exercise-induced arousal:

C: Challenge yourself.
O: Order matters.
R: Relax and receive.
E: Engage your lower abs.

In chapters 3 through 6, I expand upon each of these four principles, supplemented by exercises with photos and step-by-step instructions. In addition, all the exercises—more than thirty in all—appear in chapter 7, as do the different Coregasm Workout routines, where you can select the routine that works for you based on your skill and experience—beginner, advanced, or somewhere in between—as well as on how you happen to feel on a particular day.

Best of all, once you're armed with the knowledge hidden in the exercises, you will be able to make exciting, beneficial changes in your life. Though I suggest ways you can use exercise equipment to intensify certain exercises, you don't need fancy equipment or a gym membership to follow the C.O.R.E. Principles. Nor do you need to do all the exercises in the book—just a few will suffice! The Coregasm Workout and C.O.R.E. Principles are available to all of us. All you need is this book, an open mind, and the willingness to get sweaty. If you're ready to learn how exercise can get you in touch with your body's natural arousal and more, turn the page.

Very often, people want to know whether their chances of experiencing arousal during exercise are better if they get stronger. Here is what our research studies, to date, suggest about coregasms and strength.

STRENGTH MAY MATTER. Coregasms might be easier to achieve as people practice exercises that engage their core abdominal muscles.

CHALLENGING THE CORE MAY BE KEY. Men and boys, in general but not always, have a stronger core than women and girls. (This is just a generalization; some women have very strong abs and a strong core, more than many men.) We think this may explain why men and boys often had coregasms after quite difficult exercises such as climbing, pull-ups, and chin-ups—some of the toughest core exercises a person can do, exercises that likely asked a lot of their core, perhaps thus triggering exercise arousal or orgasm. Women, on the other hand, listed a wider range of exercises, including dancing and walking, as among those that led to an exercise-induced orgasm. The idea is that, if a person has a weaker core to begin with, it may not take as much to fatigue the muscles and then perhaps experience core arousal or orgasm.

THERE MAY BE MORE THAN ONE PATH TO EXERCISE AROUSAL/ ORGASM. People who reported orgasm or arousal from very difficult exercises (like pull-ups or chin-ups) often stated they occurred very quickly. On the other hand, people who described having orgasms or arousal from less difficult exercises, like crunches, often said it took longer to get there. Again, we keep seeing that muscular fatigue or exhaustion is a common element in coregasm. With difficult exercises, that fatigue could come quickly; with less challenging exercises, it can take more time or more reps to reach the same level of exhaustion.

WHEN DOES IT HAPPEN?

In addition to narrowing down the exercises themselves, we wanted to know *when*—at what point in the exercise—the orgasm or arousal happened and how it felt. Did it start immediately with the first or second rep? After ten reps? After a hundred? What about aerobic activities? How long into the swimming, running, or hiking did the arousal or orgasm occur? We learned that exercise arousal and orgasm almost never happen right away; it usually takes some time (fatiguing those muscles) or reps before that level of intensity is reached.

For Candace it was a matter of frequency: the more often she worked her core, the more easily her exercises led to orgasm. To the question of how many reps it takes for leg raises to trigger orgasm, she replied: "It will happen sooner the more I've been working out. So, if it is something I had been doing frequently, you know like maybe a couple of times a week, then it will take fewer than the twenty reps it would normally take."

Lisa had the opposite experience. The stronger her core abdominal muscles became, the more repetitions she had to do in order to experience orgasm during exercise. In other words, when she's not as strong, it doesn't take as many reps to fatigue her muscles, so she orgasms sooner in the process.

Aparna started going to the gym and exercising more often after gaining weight from being sedentary. She began doing ab training and weight training and experienced her first experience with coregasm doing squats with light weights (usually about five-pound hand weights). She said, "I was quite confused for a while. And then it happened again a couple of days later . . . so I Googled it."

She also asked her gynecologist whether it was all right to have an orgasm while exercising and was assured that it's completely fine. When I interviewed Aparna, she said, "[My gynecologist] just asked me how [intense the orgasm] was. I said, 'It's just like, *whoa*, kind of on a scale of 1 to 10, it's about a 5 or 6.' My doctor said, 'That's common, that's not a problem. Unless you drop the weights on the floor or you go into the *When Harry Met Sally* kind of moaning phase [in the gym], then don't worry about it.'"

Because Aparna hadn't exercised much in her life, her abs and overall core muscles were likely pretty weak. When she started doing squats, she experienced orgasm pretty quickly—after around three or four squats.

For both Lisa and Aparna, a weaker core seemed to translate to easier orgasms whereas for others, including Candace, the opposite has been true.

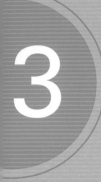**3**

The exercise orgasms usually happen during high-load experiences—either lifting weights or high-intensity hill climbs on my mountain bike.

—NATE

CHAPTER 3

C.O.R.E. PRINCIPLE 1: CHALLENGE YOURSELF

W HEN PEDALING HARD against grueling climbs, one of my favorite spin instructors often roots us on, saying, "No challenge, no change!" Though we're all about to fall off our cycles from exhaustion, we power through—and it's totally worth it. I feel strong and powerful after I've given my all to a good workout. There's something about a difficult but invigorating workout that keeps me coming back for more.

I'd like to co-opt and tweak my instructor's rallying cry to "No challenge, no coregasm." Why? Because nearly every person in our research who experienced exercise-induced arousal or orgasm did so from intense physical challenge, usually involving increased heart rate (which improves cardiovascular health), abdominal exercises, or strength training. But, as we are all different, make sure to take into account your age, health, personal history, and fitness goals when deciding how vigorously you want to exercise and the kinds of exercises you should do. You'll find assorted workout routines in chapter 7 for all fitness levels, beginner through advanced. No matter what experience and fitness you bring to the mat, there's a path for you. As with any exercise program, be sure to consult a doctor or nurse before initiating a new exercise regimen.

Assuming you're physically ready to get started and get sweaty, you can push yourself by pursuing the following approaches—noted briefly here, then expanded upon just below.

ACTIVATE YOUR "ON" SWITCH. On days you'd like to explore exercise arousal, trigger your sympathetic nervous system—your "fight or flight" response—with intense exercise. No light, easy breezy pace for you—or me! (More on that below.)

ADD CARDIO. The best sympathetic nervous system activator is intense cardio, especially just before heading into a core- or ab-focused workout. This could be brisk walking or jogging, working the treadmill, biking, dancing, or taking a spin or step class—basically, any activity that's guaranteed to get your blood pumping.

WORK A LITTLE HARDER. Once you've added cardio to your routine, intensify your effort. Look for opportunities to add a little more guts for a lot more glory. If you're walking or running, consider charging up some hills. If you're on an indoor cardio machine, choose a more challenging program than usual.

ADD RESISTANCE THROUGH WEIGHTS. There are several ways to make your core workouts more challenging, such as adding weight lifting or resistance training to your routine. Or, if you're already doing that, then challenge yourself with heavier weights, including your own body weight, as with pull-ups or chin-ups.

INCREASE YOUR REPS. You can also challenge yourself by increasing your reps, especially by adding more reps to your sets, and reducing your rest periods in between.

INCREASE EXERCISE FREQUENCY. Frequent workouts help you maintain and build core strength over time. Unless you already work out almost every day, try adding one more session to your week, or add five to ten minutes to your total workout time; then, in time, add an additional workout or an extra few minutes. Keep challenging yourself.

Now, let's take a closer look at each of these modifications so you can choose the ones that are right for you.

ACTIVATE YOUR "ON" SWITCH

Activating your sympathetic nervous system, or "on" switch, may help you reach arousal more easily when you shift to core exercises.

Did you know you have an "on" switch? You do; it's called the sympathetic nervous system (SNS), which is what triggers our "fight or flight" response to particular environments. The SNS can be activated by anxiety—such as you might experience watching a scary movie, riding a rollercoaster, or crossing a shaky bridge—or even by getting overly excited rooting for your favorite team. Consider, for example, this description of the circus of ancient Rome:

> *It was often said: "The great spectacle at the circus is not the games but the spectators." The games were the great emotional outlet for the mob and they made the most of it. During a race the crowd literally went mad. Women collapsed or had sexual orgasms. Men bit themselves, tore their clothes, did mad dances, bet until they ran out of money.... One man fainted when the white team fell behind.... Travelers approaching Rome could hear the roar of triumph when the race was over before they could see the city towers. [They] stood up in the stands drumming with their fists on the back of people in the seats before them and screaming hysterically: "Kill! Kill! Kill!" Even before the games started, smart young men could spot women who would give way to this madness and make a point of sitting next to them.*
> —DANIEL P. MANNIX, *THOSE ABOUT TO DIE*

As the above quotation so colorfully describes, and as numerous studies have demonstrated, activation of the SNS can enhance women's sexual arousal. When our SNS is activated, our heart rate and blood pressure increase. Our breath quickens. And one pretty reliable trigger for activating our SNS response is intense exercise, especially cardio exercise.

ADD CARDIO

Adding 30–60 minutes of intense cardio before moving directly into core exercises can increase the likelihood of exercise-induced arousal and orgasm.

Time and again, women we interviewed told us that doing cardio first mattered to their exercise arousal or orgasms. And of the women keeping exercise diaries, many of those who began experiencing arousal did so by doing cardio first, then moving directly to a core abdominal workout with minimal break in between. Aparna told us the following:

> I think that my muscles are already warmed up so there's arousal without me knowing, but in my mind that doesn't figure as arousal because I'm just working out. There have been times when I haven't worked out much on the treadmill or the elliptical, and then, in spite of doing more crunches, . . . orgasm hasn't happened then. But when I actually work out for the full one hour on the treadmill or elliptical first, that's when orgasm usually happens.

One woman experienced arousal from crunches only if she'd done some kind of aerobic activity just before—be it walking her dog for close to an hour, riding her bike home from work, or doing a cardio workout in her living room. Another reported she surprised herself with her first coregasm by moving from an intense stair-climbing workout right into working her abs with planks.

As we gathered more data, the pattern became clear that doing cardio first—and doing it for a significant length of time, often between half an hour and an hour—strongly influences women's exercise arousal and orgasm.

That a lengthy cardio workout was needed for many to reach arousal leads us to the next point: the role of muscle exhaustion in triggering the arousal response. One study participant shared that she runs "beyond the point of exhaustion," tensing her leg, stomach, and bottom muscles as she runs. Many women and men found that intensifying their workouts, to the point that they exhausted their bodies and fatigued their muscles, was key to inducing arousal.

WORK A LITTLE HARDER

When you're ready to experiment with exercise-induced arousal, push yourself a little harder or further than before.

However you enjoy exercising, you can find ways to challenge yourself. Increase the incline or speed on the treadmill. Spin or bike up tougher inclines. Alternate between walking and jogging. Add sprints to your runs. Try harder machines at the gym. Take a more advanced cardio class. Intensify your effort.

Although what we're sharing here applies to a great number of women, that doesn't mean everyone responds the same—far from it.

Among the women who reached arousal during ab work, some found that cardio wasn't a *necessary* precursor to exercise arousal or orgasm—but it often helped. For example, one woman told us that if she hadn't done cardio first, it might take her several minutes to reach coregasm during her ab workout; whereas if she had done cardio first, she could coregasm within thirty seconds. This resonates with sex orgasms: the more aroused people feel leading into sex, the more likely they will orgasm.

And while most women can reach arousal only during core exercises and generally after doing cardio first, some women experienced coreorgasm *during cardio*—but only after a significant stretch of activity. I don't think we had a single woman report that she experienced orgasm in the first few minutes of cardio work, even if it was strenuous.

As you move through the Coregasm Workout and try it out for yourself, the most important thing is to pay attention to your own personal experience of exercise and arousal. You may learn important things about yourself and develop an awareness of your body and its sensations that can help you feel more connected to your body and better able to translate these new discoveries to your sex life.

If you're into yoga, try sinking deeper into poses, or holding them for the maximum time your instructor recommends. One woman noted she reached coregasms only in hot yoga classes when she'd worked especially hard.

For some, training harder meant running or biking uphill; Kelly in particular found uphill cycling worked best for her. Some who've experienced arousal from spin class noticed it occurred soon after a particularly intense hill climb.

Sprinting can also be an effective intensifier: for reasons we don't fully understand, brief periods of acceleration can help trigger arousal. Perhaps it activates the sympathetic nervous system. Or it concerns a physical mechanism: the act of acceleration—from jogging to running, from standing still to sprinting—shifts our organs, muscles, ligaments, and nerves in ways that possibly induce arousal. In other research, some people

Note that working a little harder doesn't mean you can't ever take it easy or enjoy leisurely exercise. In fact, rest and recovery are important components of any exercise program or training. Be sure to stretch after your core exercises or weight lifting. Wrap up a tough swim with a few comfortable laps and then some stretches. Finish a run with a few minutes of leisurely walking. These wind-down approaches help your heart rate return to normal, which is an important part of recovery.

With weight training in particular, rest days (with no exercise) or days with easier workouts are essential for giving your muscles time to recover. You want to avoid "overtraining" yourself.

even say they have orgasms from other kinds of "acceleration activities," like driving up and down hills in a car, speeding, or riding on a rollercoaster.

Sometimes, the moment when we want to give up is exactly when we should keep going. This is often as true in fitness as it is in our day-to-day lives, including work, school, and going through difficult times with our families and friends. Stick with it. Intensify your effort. You can do it!

There is no one "right" way to exercise—or to recover—that fits everyone. People have different fitness and recovery needs based on their age, health, personal history, and fitness goals. Bikini bodybuilders have different fitness needs than professional volleyball players, who, in turn, have different fitness needs than people who are training for their first 5K run or walk. You (and your doctor, physical therapist, coach, and/or personal trainer) will know your fitness needs the best.

I believe that balance in our lives and in our workouts is key. Rest days help our bodies and our muscles recover, which is critical. Make sure to honor your body and its needs through rest and recovery!

ADD RESISTANCE THROUGH WEIGHTS

In addition to helping build muscle and burning calories, adding resistance builds a solid foundation for exercise arousal and orgasm.

When we exercise, certain primary muscles do much of the work. When our muscles get fatigued, or when a movement is particularly complex, other nearby muscles get "recruited" to help share the load. One theory we have about coregasm is that some of these nearby muscles are those that are closer to, or even attach to, the lower pelvic or genital area. So it's when we've pushed ourselves to the point of fatigue that the nearby muscles are most likely to help out—and when we're more likely to experience arousal.

In the next two sections we'll discuss two excellent means of exhausting the muscles: increasing duration (by adding reps, which we'll cover soon), and increasing load.

You can increase the load you expect your muscles to bear by adding weights or resistance to your workout routine. Or, if you already do strength training, challenge your muscles to work harder by choosing a slightly heavier weight. These were the methods that helped some of our study participants to experience arousal. One woman wrote:

> *The only time I experienced an orgasm while exercising was using a machine that involved bringing a weighted apparatus downward from above my head to shoulder height using my arms, abdominal/core muscles, and shoulders. This seemed to occur when I was using a heavier weight than what I used typically. I became aroused and climaxed very quickly over the course of 3 or 4 repetitions. The stimulation seemed to be coming from the use/strain of my abdominal muscles.*

Another woman experienced arousal from push-ups. She wrote, "Mostly this occurred when I'd reached a point where I was starting to become fatigued, and it felt like every muscle was flexing to keep me stabilized." Again, this idea, that certain muscles do the primary work but other nearby muscles help out, may be related to some women's experiences of arousing or orgasmic exercise.

One woman, a personal trainer, tends to respond mostly to pretty intense exercises; all the same, the point is that she challenges herself:

> *I've experienced orgasm a handful of times with heavy 45-degree, plate-loaded leg presses, but almost* every single time *with hanging leg raises. I get past a threshold of being completely miserable and wanting to stop, but continuing with*

the exercise anyway. I have to squeeze really hard to keep going and then I feel it building and I can just keep going and going and going.

People sometimes think of weight lifting as not being an aerobic or cardiovascular exercise. However, if you're working hard while you're lifting weights—if you're choosing challenging weights and doing lots of reps—then a strength workout will get your heart rate up, which can both build muscle and burn calories, and of course increase your chances of exercise arousal.

INCREASE YOUR REPS

Increasing the number of reps you do will both make for a more demanding workout and make exercise-induced arousal more likely.

Many of us were taught to exercise in sets. So, if you set out to do 30 crunches, you'd do them in, say, three sets of 10 crunches, with a break between sets. This is a common approach to fitness that allows time to recover between sets. If you prefer to exercise in sets, then consider increasing the number of reps per set. For example, rather than three sets of 10, why not try three sets of 12 or 15? That's one way to challenge yourself.

Some opt to work toward exhaustion without breaks in between, an approach we've found can increase the chances of feeling aroused while exercising. In fitness circles, some people describe this as continuous exercise (reps done all in a row, without stopping in between), which is different from discontinuous training (exercise done in sets, with breaks in between).

A study published in the *Journal of Strength and Conditioning Research* tested both approaches; it found that continuous training (going all at once, rather than sets) was more of a challenge. And remember: no challenge, no change! And no challenge, no coregasm!

If you are up for a challenge, and it fits with your fitness and health goals, you might see whether adding more reps—or doing your reps all at once (rather than in sets)—makes a difference for you.

Also, you can vary the way you use weights with your reps. Some people prefer to do more reps with lighter weights; others do fewer reps with heavier weights. There are also ways to combine these strategies. For example, you could:

COREGASM 101 CARE TO DANCE?

A number of women in our studies said they experienced arousal or orgasm from dancing. They often specified it was the movements themselves, not just the fact that they felt sexy at the time, that induced their arousal. Andrea wrote:

> The dance class I take is a rather sexual activity, with a lot of hip movement, booty shaking, and overall sexiness. When I'm shaking, rotating, gyrating, it feels so sexy I can't help but be aroused. I also enjoy thinking about the fantastic effects these movements will have on my body and my sex life, and how sexy I'll look when I dance. These thoughts, combined with the movement, lead to sexual pleasure.

Dancing to music, even at home on your own, is a great way to feel sexy and confident—regardless of whether you'll be meeting up with someone later. And of course dancing with a partner, whether at a club or in the kitchen, can make for fun and sensuous foreplay.

There are great exercise benefits to dancing as well, including the increased heart rate achieved with cardio work. And if while dancing you engage your core, especially those lower abs, you just might get an extra boost of physical arousal to boot!

Do sets that get progressively harder (such as three sets of 10 biceps curls, where the first set of 10 is done with light weights, the second set of 10 with medium weights, and the third set with heavier weights);

or

Do sets that get progressively easier (starting with heavier weights and finishing with lighter weights).

Keep in mind that all changes take time. The first few times you do your crunches or leg lifts all at once, or with more reps, you may not feel any difference. It takes time to build core strength. In addition, it can take practice to learn to be mindful of your bodily sensations and to learn to connect with feelings of arousal, particularly if those feelings haven't previously been part of your exercise experience. Try to be gentle and compassionate with yourself.

COREGASM 101 PRACTICE SAFER COREGASMS!

One woman I interviewed described frequently having orgasms while she runs on the treadmill, and these orgasms are associated with her momentarily zoning out. Though she's never fallen off the treadmill, she has had the occasional experience of a close call. Having the cord that connects from the machine to her wrist has helped her stop the machine when her pace changed as her orgasm started, and has been a saving grace in each instance.

Most of the time, experiencing arousal or orgasm through exercise seems to go off without a hitch. It doesn't feel sexual to most people who experience it—and so it doesn't even look or feel awkward to them or to those around them. It's just a bodily experience.

If you're worried about losing control, though, you may not want to try exercise arousal or orgasm with exercises that involve throwing a medicine ball in the air, let alone climbing a rope or pole and being suspended midair! Instead, Russian twists (see chapter 6) and other exercises that involve holding on to a ball might be safer choices, as might planks or bicycle crunches or any number of other exercises that keep you grounded on the floor. If you're experimenting with exercise arousal or orgasm on a treadmill, you might want to attach the cord from the machine to your shorts, which—if pulled—shuts the machine completely off.

INCREASE EXERCISE FREQUENCY

When you increase exercise frequency and strength, you're better equipped to reach the thresholds most people need to achieve arousal and coregasm.

When I work out more regularly, and when I include more of the core exercises from chapter 7, I'm more likely to experience arousal. Why? Probably because I've built up enough strength to reach the thresholds our research suggests make it easier to experience arousal and coregasm. And I'm not the only one—not by any means.

Rose gets aroused from doing pull-ups. And she works out frequently: she's strong enough to do enough pull-ups to the point of arousal and even coregasm.

Both Steven, whom I mentioned earlier, and Jayson feel that their coregasmic abilities are tied to their strength or muscle tone—for which they exercise often so as to maintain that strength and experience arousal. Another man wrote, "The strength or

COREGASM 101 A NOTE TO PERSONAL TRAINERS EVERYWHERE

I hope it's abundantly clear by now that exercise arousal and orgasm are not all that un-common. About 10 percent of women and men have had orgasms while exercising, and many more have felt aroused while exercising. So what does this have to do with you? If you work as a personal trainer, you may find yourself working with clients who prefer not to do certain exercises. You may feel it's your job to push them to overcome their reluctance for the sake of their health and fitness.

The thing is, there are any number of reasons clients might feel reluctant to do some-thing, and they're all valid: injury, pain, or discomfort; embarrassment about particular moves; or even simply not enjoying a particular exercise. And allow me to offer an addi-tional possibility: clients may be reluctant to experience exercise-induced orgasm in the company of others. So, if a client chooses not to do an exercise, please respect that choice without probing too deeply. The choice should be theirs, not yours.

tone of my stomach muscles seems to have a direct bearing on my ability to achieve a coregasm." And we've also heard from both women and men whose exercise-induced arousal in their younger years revived after they got back in shape—in other words, after a period of irregular or infrequent exercise, it was only when they started exercising reg-ularly again that their arousal returned.

One woman described her orgasm and arousal as a sort of cycle, with each motivat-ing the other: "Sometimes I use the arousal as motivation to keep going, or as a reward for myself when I've finished what I set out to do. Or, sometimes, if I see someone in bet-ter shape I think to myself, *You may look better, but I'm having more fun!*" Remember: ex-ercise arousal and orgasms may not be about sex in the traditional sense, and they don't feel quite the same as orgasms from sex, but that doesn't mean they don't feel good!

4 It's after the cardio. I always do cardio then [legs, abs, or weights], and so I think the cardio gets me going; gets my heart rate up, gets my adrenaline pumping a little bit, and that can play a factor sometimes. . . . For legs, I do four sets of 40 lunges or three sets of 50 squats. . . . It's very common for me to feel aroused [during my leg routine] but not so very common for me to orgasm. [When I feel aroused], it's in the last set [of squats or lunges].

—DANIELLE

CHAPTER 4

C.O.R.E. PRINCIPLE 2: ORDER MATTERS

VERY OFTEN I read magazine or website articles about coregasms that focus solely on the specific *types* of exercises linked with orgasm. As a result, they recommend that the reader do leg lifts on the Captain's/Roman Chair, for example—but there's more to it than that, as you know by now. If feeling aroused or orgasmic was as simple as hopping on a Captain's/Roman Chair and doing a few leg raises, there wouldn't be much mystery to it at all. It doesn't work that way.

How people order, or sequence, their exercises matters, and in unique, important ways, say most people who have participated in our research. This is similar to sex.

When it comes to sex, most people have some kind of routine: an order they follow to experience the most pleasure. This applies as much to "sex for one" as it does to partnered sex. For many couples, the routine often involves kissing, taking off clothes, erotic touch, possibly oral sex, intercourse, and then sleep—in that order. Sex researchers call these routines "sexual scripts," and have found them to be highly predictable, as much for individuals as for couples. Of course, different couples have different scripts. Even one person's script with a former partner can differ greatly from the script followed with one's current partner.

Order matters with exercise arousal too: how people sequence their exercises strongly influences their arousal in ways that are unique to them. We've already seen examples of this: while one woman's exercise arousal or orgasm requires leg lifts to the point of fatigue, another woman relies on pull-ups. To follow, I share some of what we learned, with tips on how you can apply these lessons to discovering your own go-to arousal routine.

ORDER IS UNIQUE TO EVERYONE

Having an ordered routine facilitates exercise arousal, but it requires practice and modification to discover what sequence of exercises works best for you.

You may recall that none of the women in our coregasm diary research had experienced exercise-induced arousal prior to our study. On the other hand, the women from our earlier interview studies were coregasm pros. As a result, they knew which exercise routines reliably worked for them.

We shared earlier how Shannon reaches coregasm through running: "I generally get fairly aroused when I've run more than a couple miles. After that I can often orgasm by contracting my pelvic muscles several times in quick succession. Occasionally I'll orgasm just from running—without even trying. But if I feel that coming on I can usually stop it by slowing down or changing my gait."

Learning what your body responds to with exercise can provide insight into your body's particular responses to sex. Like Shannon, some women noticed that squeezing their ab or pelvic muscles during exercises induced arousal; often squeezing in the same manner during sex proved fruitful. In an earlier chapter, Jane noted it was easier to contract these muscles during sex because with intercourse she had "something to squeeze."

You may remember Rose, who stays fit in order to be strong enough to pull off the coregasms she gets from pull-ups. Through trial and error she determined the particular routine that worked for her. Because the pull-ups were so intense, requiring a great deal of energy, she purposely didn't do any tiring exercise first, saving her strength for about nine pull-ups. Then, toward the end, she'd hang on the bar and pull her knees toward her chest, which intensified the pleasurable sensations.

So, essentially, having a personal routine—knowing which activities, and in which order, will produce results for you—can be a pretty reliable route to exercise arousal. If you already have an exercise routine, it would likely take only minor modifications to help you tap into your arousal. To follow you'll also find some routines that have worked for other women; perhaps they'll work for you too.

COREGASM 101 FOR ALL ROUTINES

If you begin to feel arousal, try to notice about how many reps or sets of a certain exercise it takes before the arousal kicks in. And, as pleasant as the arousal can feel, remember: the exercises are just a way to connect with your body. Don't neglect to do non-arousing exercises too. For total wellness, it's important to use all your major muscle groups when you exercise, and not just the ones that make you feel tingly!

Lyla's Gym Cardio Routine

1. Begin with 30–45 minutes of intense cardio, such as running on the treadmill or using the elliptical machine.

   After you've been exercising for a while, pay attention to any bodily sensations that feel like arousal to you. (In order to intensify her feelings of arousal, Lyla listens to music with strong bass beats.)

   To challenge yourself during your cardio work, try increasing the incline or alternating between 1 minute at a moderate pace and 30 seconds at an intense pace.

2. Transition into a core routine. For example:

   cat/cow
   bridge
   prone plank or supine plank
   bicycle crunches
   leg raises
   push-ups
   superman
   (Details for these exercises appear below.)

3. Make sure to stretch before calling it a day.

This routine is also a good place to start for spine health, as exercises like cat/cow, bridge, and plank are some of the most highly recommended for beginning a core workout because they can serve as gentle wake-ups for your spine.

CAT/COW

The cat/cow posture is common to many yoga classes, and is sometimes used in childhood dance classes. It's a great warm-up since it gently moves the spine.

1. Begin on all fours in a "tabletop" position. Your hands should be directly beneath your shoulders, your knees directly beneath your hips. Your spine should be in a neutral position—in a relatively straight line from your head to your hips. It may help to think of having a long neck (*pictured, top*). Your gaze should be toward the floor.

2. On an inhale, move into cow pose by lifting your sitting bones up, gently lifting your chest and chin, and gazing toward the ceiling. Some people choose to curl their toes under as well. Try to move slowly and gently, with your neck the last part to move (*pictured, bottom left*).

3. On an exhale, move into cat by rounding your spine, tucking your tailbone, and dropping your head; your gaze should be toward the floor or your navel (*pictured, bottom right*).

4. Alternate between cow pose and cat pose about 10 times in slow, fluid movements. Be sure to consistently inhale for cow pose and exhale for cat pose.

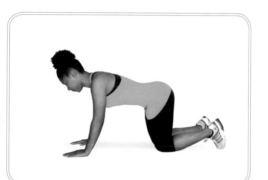

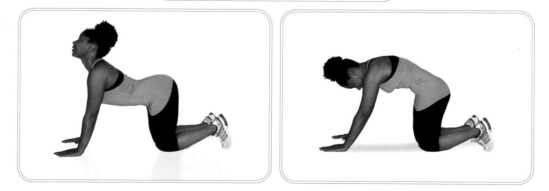

BRIDGE

Bridge is another pose that's gentle on the spine, which makes it ideal both toward the beginning and toward the end of a workout session.

1. Lie on your back with your knees bent and your arms on the floor alongside your body (*pictured, left*). Your feet should be flat on the floor with your heels close to your sitting bones. Palms can be flat or facing up.

2. On an exhale, press your feet and arms into the floor as you squeeze your buttocks and core abdominal muscles, thus lifting your hips off the floor (*pictured, right*). Your thighs should be parallel and your knees should be over your heels.

3. Try to maintain core engagement (continue squeezing) for as long as you hold this pose.

4. If you are comfortable in the pose and would like to take it deeper, clasp your hands together on the mat underneath your body.

5. Stay in the pose for at least 5 breath cycles. As you become more comfortable in the pose, try to build up to holding the bridge for about 10 breath cycles.

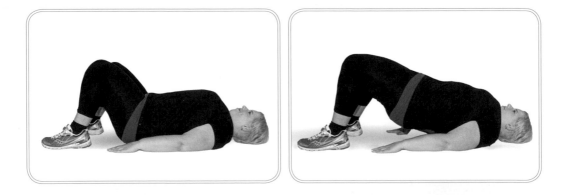

PRONE PLANK

Modeled on the push-up, plank exercises have become very popular in recent years, and are often considered an essential part of core fitness programs. Though planks may look simple, they require constant, active engagement of a number of core muscles, which can help build a strong core.

1. Start by lying facedown on the floor with your palms touching the floor directly beneath your shoulders. Your core should be tight.

2. Push/lift yourself into a bent-knee push-up or a standard push-up.

   BENT-KNEE VARIATION: Your knees remain touching the floor, your calves and feet in the air behind you. This variation can make planks easier to incorporate into your workout since it requires your core to support less of your body weight. Your body should be in a straight line from your head to your knees.

   STANDARD (STRAIGHT) LEG: Keep your legs straight with the balls of your feet on the floor. They can be planted wide apart (which is easier) or closer together (which is more challenging).

3. Your body should form a relatively straight line, either from your head to your knees (bent-knee variation) or from your head to your feet (straight-leg variation). Keeping your abs stiff will make it easier to stay in plank, so try to keep your back flat, pulling your belly button toward your spine (*as pictured*).

4. For more muscle engagement, squeeze your glutes and engage your quads as if you're drawing your kneecaps up toward your thighs.

5. Breathe in and out.

6. If you're new to plank, try to stay in the plank position for about 10 seconds. As you build strength and comfort, work up to holding for 30 seconds, then for 1 minute. Some people work toward holding planks for several minutes. Do what feels right for you!

(continued) ▶

Ways to Challenge Yourself

- Advance from bent-knee to standard plank.

- Bring your feet closer together.

- Hold the position longer—even up to 4 minutes, if you can!

- Lift one leg (or one arm) off the ground.

- Instead of having your hands on the floor, plank with your forearms and elbows on the floor. Your forearms should completely touch the floor, with your elbows directly beneath your shoulders.

- Plank on a large exercise ball instead of on the ground, resting your forearms on the ball. You should feel your body working to balance and stabilize itself.

(For the supine plank, see page 103.)

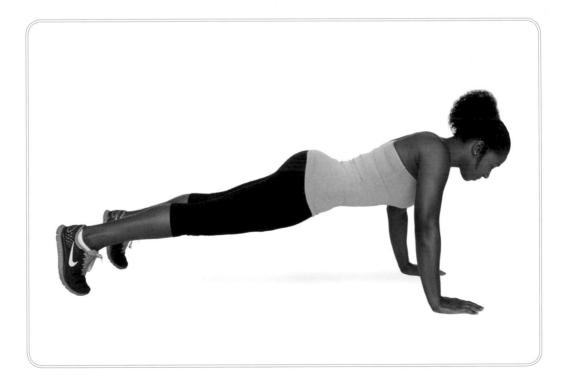

BICYCLE CRUNCHES

Bicycle crunches are a common core exercise that effectively engages several abdominal muscles. They can be arousal-inducing as well; bicycle crunches are some women's primary coregasmic exercise.

1. Lie on your back with your knees bent and feet planted on the floor, about hip-width apart.

2. Start by drawing your right knee toward your chest and straightening your left leg as you crunch forward, drawing your left elbow toward your right knee (*as pictured*). Your left elbow and shoulder blade should come just a few inches off the floor.

3. Now reverse the move: straighten your right leg and draw your left knee toward your chest as you crunch forward, drawing your right elbow toward your left knee. This time your right elbow and shoulder blade will come just a few inches off the floor.

4. Keep alternating sides. Aim for at least 10 crunches in each direction; eventually, try to work up to 20 to 30 on each side, or to the point of muscle fatigue.

Tips

- Do not pull on your neck and do not push your head with your hands. Your abs should be doing the work here.

- Try to focus on a slow and controlled movement.

Ways to Challenge Yourself

- If you've developed a strong core and can keep going with good form, try continuing bicycle crunches to the point of fatigue. Some women do as many as 50 to 100 crunches per side!

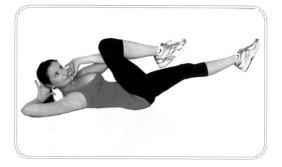

LEG RAISES

Leg raises—whether done lying on the floor, as pictured here, or on a Captain's Chair/Roman Chair at the gym—commonly lead to arousal for some women. Leg raises on the floor are easier and safer than those done on a Captain's Chair/Roman Chair, which are best attempted with a trainer to ensure proper form.

1. Lying on your back, lift your legs in the air until they are perpendicular to your body, about a 90-degree angle (*pictured, left*).

2. While keeping your abs tight and your navel pulled in toward your spine, very slowly lower your legs toward the floor in a smooth and controlled motion (*pictured, right*). Press your back into the floor while lowering your legs down toward the floor, but stop before your feet reach the floor.

3. Lift your legs back to the starting position and repeat. Aim to do 10 reps at first; over time, work to complete 20–30 reps.

Tips

- Make sure your lower back stays on the floor. If you feel your lower back arching or coming off the floor, don't lower your legs any farther. That may be a good stopping place for you.

- As you continue to do core exercises more regularly, you may develop enough strength to eventually lower your legs closer to the floor.

Ways to Challenge Yourself

- As you grow stronger and build endurance, it may take more reps to get you to the point of fatigue—perhaps as many as 50–100 leg raises.

- To mix it up and keep it interesting, do single leg raises instead of lifting and lowering both at once.

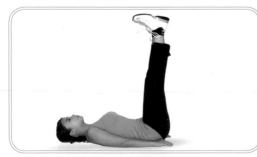 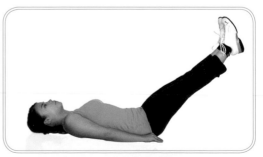

PUSH-UPS

"Drop and give me 10!" Many of us first tried doing some form of push-up when we were kids. A push-up is a classic core exercise that also engages various muscles in the chest and back. For some, they can also induce arousal.

To follow, we offer steps for the two most common push-ups: the push-up from the knee and the standard push-up. Freddie (*pictured*) is demonstrating the standard push-up on an overturned balance trainer.

1. Start by lying facedown on the floor with your palms touching the floor directly beneath your shoulders. Your core should be tight.

   BENT-KNEE VARIATION: Bend your knees so your calves and feet are in the air behind you. Your knees remain touching the floor.

2. With your feet (or knees) still touching the floor, and keeping your eyes focused on the floor, in a slow and controlled motion straighten your arms to push/lift yourself into a push-up (*pictured, left*). Note that your body should be in a straight line from your head to your feet (or from your head to your knees if you're doing the bent-knee variation).

3. In a slow and controlled motion, bend your elbows so that you lower your chest and chin close to the floor without fully reaching it (*pictured, right*). Make sure to keep your abs tight (drawing your navel toward your spine) throughout the push-up. Keep your body in a straight line.

4. Repeat the process, aiming for a few push-ups, if possible.

(continued) ▶

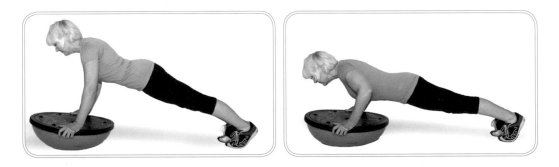

Tips

- At first you may be able to do just a few push-ups—or even just one. That's okay! Push-ups are a difficult exercise that uses your body weight for resistance.

- Over time you can build up to 10, then 20, then 30 or more.

Ways to Challenge Yourself

- Graduate from knee push-ups to standard push-ups.

- Once you're comfortable with standard push-ups, adjust how wide apart you plant your feet: wide apart is easier; closer together is more challenging.

- For a change of pace or to work on your balance, try push-ups on a balance trainer, as Freddie (*pictured*) is doing.

SUPERMAN

Superman is good for your core, glutes, hamstrings, and lower back. Many people neglect lower back exercises, but they are an important part of core training. Plus, given its motion of squeezing and tensing the body, Superman is also an exercise that some find particularly arousing.

1. Start by lying on your stomach with your arms extended in front of you and your legs stretched behind you, feet apart (*pictured, top*).

2. Keeping your arms and legs straight and your core fully engaged and tight, all at once raise your arms, chest, and feet a few inches off the floor by stretching your arms out and squeezing your butt and thighs together (*pictured, bottom*). Continue to breathe in and out.

3. Try to hold this pose for 10 seconds at first, then release and relax. Try to repeat 2–3 times.

Tips

- At first you may be able to lift your upper and lower body only an inch or two off the ground. That's okay. With practice you can increase your core strength, and over time may be able to lift higher.

Ways to Challenge Yourself

- Over time, work toward holding this pose for 30–60 seconds, then release.

- Or, rather than holding it for a length of time, increase your reps, up to 20–30, but holding for just 1 or 2 seconds each.

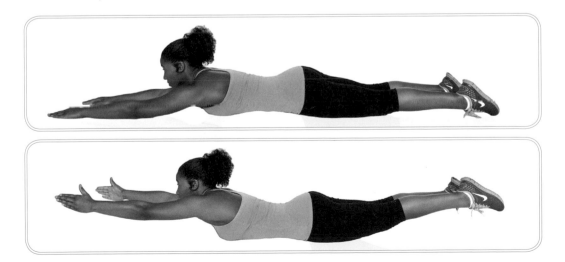

Maureen's Core Routine

As with all the routines, keep attentive to your body's response, whether signs of arousal or just generally pleasant feelings. And if you feel discomfort or pain, listen to your body! Ask your healthcare provider or personal trainer questions about your own personal health or fitness needs.

1. Walk briskly, or run, for 30–45 minutes. Try to focus on keeping your core engaged, drawing your belly button toward your spine. For better posture, keep your shoulders pressed back. Then transition quickly into your core workout, with little (if any) break in between.

2. Transition into bridge position (*see page 58*). Hold for 30 seconds. Relax for 10 seconds. Then repeat twice (for a total of three 30-second bridges).

   When you're in the bridge position, focus on engaging your core, making your abs feel contracted and stiff.

   You might also try squeezing and releasing your pelvic floor muscles as you would with Kegel exercises.

3. Bicycle crunches (*see page 61*). Maureen does 40 in a row rather than in sets. If you do these in sets, try to rest only as long as you need to in between.

4. Stability ball pass (*details below*). Again, do what you can. Push your body toward fatigue.

5. Superman (*see page 65*) or the Swimmer (*details below*). Next do an exercise, like Superman or the swimmer, that targets your back muscles, as they're also an important part of your core.

6. Finish with stretches.

STABILITY BALL PASS

This is another fun core exercise, though it takes a little coordination. Be patient with yourself.

1. With a large exercise ball in your hands, begin by lying on the floor with your arms stretched above your head and your feet shoulder-width apart (*pictured, top*).

2. Keeping your limbs outstretched, lift your arms and legs to meet, with the ball in your hands now above your body. "Hugging" the ball on either side with your feet, transfer/pass the ball from your hands to your feet (*pictured, middle*).

3. With the ball now secured by your feet, lower your arms and legs back toward the floor (*pictured, bottom*).

4. Repeat the process in reverse, returning the ball to your hands.

5. Try for at least 10 reps of passing the ball to your feet and returning it to your hands.

Tips

- Work to press your lower back toward the floor with this exercise. If you feel your lower back arching, don't lower your arms and legs quite so far.

Ways to Challenge Yourself

- Repeat at least 20 times or until fatigued. Some people love this exercise and do as many as 40 or more reps. Maybe you will too!

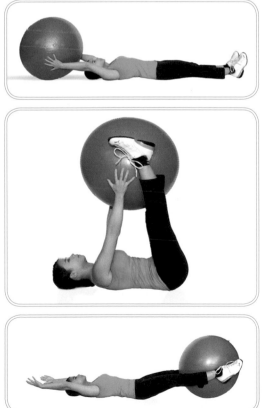

SWIMMER

The swimmer is another core exercise that is particularly beneficial for the backside of the body: glutes, hamstrings, and lower back.

1. Start by lying on your stomach with your arms stretched above your head and your legs straight.

2. Keeping your limbs straight, simultaneously lift your chest and left arm and your right leg at least several inches off the floor (*as pictured*). Aim for keeping your movements fluid and your breathing steady.

3. Switch to working the opposite limbs: lift your chest and right arm and your left leg at least several inches off the floor.

4. Continue alternating sides, breathing and fluidly moving your limbs as if you were swimming.

5. Try to do at least 10 on each side, building up to 20–30 per side.

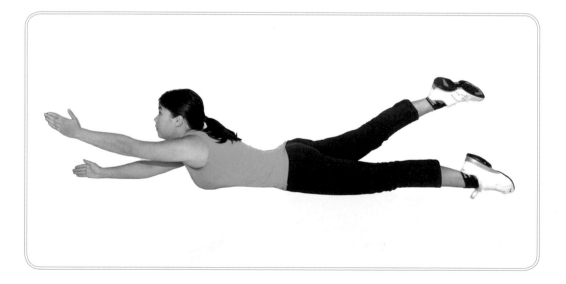

Rose's Upper-Body Strength-Building Routine

Most people find unassisted pull-ups difficult. Your gym may have an assisted pull-up machine, which is great for building upper body strength. When you're done with this pull-up routine, move into your normal weight-lifting routine, cardio exercises, or the Coregasm Workout core exercises throughout this book.

1. Begin your pull-ups: hold on to the bar above you, your palms facing either direction. Slowly pull yourself up so that your head rises above the bar.

2. Do as many pull-ups as you can. This may be only one or two to begin with. Over time, you can build strength and add more reps. Pay attention to your bodily sensations; if you notice any arousal, note where it originates. (For many women, exercise arousal begins in the lower abs.)

3. As you approach muscular fatigue and feel your ab muscles start to quiver, take a cue from Rose and slowly bring your knees toward your chest, further engaging your core muscles. Then slowly lower yourself down.

THE DYNAMICS OF THE "CARRY-OVER EFFECT"

Exercise-induced arousal isn't about finding one magical exercise; it's about noticing patterns in your exercises, and how they all work together.

A woman in the diary study noted that sometimes her arousal "carried over," as she put it, from one exercise to the next. In other words, once her arousal was kicked into gear through one exercise, that arousal was more easily or more quickly accessed in subsequent exercises—as long as the exercises were challenging and engaged the lower abdominal muscles. And she wasn't the only one to notice this: several of the diaries described similar experiences—enough that I dubbed this the "carry-over effect."

Here's a good example of it in practice, taken from one of the study diaries:

- Biked for an hour at the gym (very intensely).

- Did two sets of 25 crunches on an exercise ball; after about 20 crunches, started to feel aroused.

- Did 50 regular crunches on the floor—all at once, rather than in sets; after about 15 crunches arousal increased.

- Did 3 planks but didn't notice any arousal.

- Ended with two sets of 15 jackknife ab exercises; felt moderate arousal again after 12 jackknives.

You might have also noticed that, with each new exercise, she felt the arousal earlier and earlier: first after 20 crunches on the exercise ball, then after 15 crunches on the floor, and next after 12 jackknives. However, when she next transitioned to arm pullovers, her arousal decreased dramatically.

So how does the carry-over effect work? Most likely it has to do with the muscle fatigue we feel if we continue exercising the same muscles until we feel our body just can't do any more, or can't maintain the same vigor. Remember: one of our theories is that exercise-induced arousal and orgasm may come about because of the way nearby muscles join in to help out the fatigued muscles—particularly as some of these "helper" muscles may be in or around the genitals and the nerve pathways to orgasm. If you want to understand your own patterns, routines, and carry-over effect, keeping an exercise diary is an excellent place to start.

COREGASM 101   MINDY'S CARRY-OVER EFFECT

"The feeling is slightly pleasant in the beginning but as I do more sets, and strain the muscles more, the feeling intensifies and ends with an orgasm. The sensation becomes more and more intense every time I lift my legs. I do sets of 20 reps, with a short break in between. The first set starts out with nothing and ends with slight pleasure; the second set starts where the first left off and builds up very quickly. I will normally orgasm toward the end of the second set, sometimes halfway through the third set. It definitely feels like a friction orgasm from the inside, not the outside from my clothes. Every lower abdomen workout I do gives me pleasure, but the Captain's Chair is the only one that makes me orgasm."

—MINDY

THE VALUE OF AN EXERCISE DIARY

Keeping an exercise diary can help you stay motivated and focused while also tracking your patterns of arousal.

Keeping an exercise diary does more than just serve as a list reminding you of which exercises to do. By tracking which exercises increase your arousal and to what degree, you'll be able to monitor your progress. In reviewing your diary entries you'll likely notice patterns regarding which exercises induce arousal—and in what order, and for what duration, etc.—and whether you experienced any carry-over effect. These pertinent data will help you tailor the exercise routine that works best for you.

For example, you might notice that every time you do bicycle crunches, your arousal kicks in; but when you switch to leg raises, it goes away. That's helpful information, providing valuable feedback on how you can move your body to enhance arousal. Paying such close attention to your body and its responses is a form of mindfulness, which has been shown to help women enhance their sexual arousal in the bedroom, too.

To that end, you could track how or whether your workouts influence your sex life, again looking for patterns. Do you have better sex on days you have an intense workout? Or maybe on days when you work out with your partner? After a fun evening dance class? Or after a relaxing morning yoga class?

If you'd like to track your data online, visit us at www.TheCoregasmWorkout.com and follow the links. You'll find diary templates both at this site and in this book's appendix. You'll also find a sample marked-up diary page on the following pages.

So let's walk through how the diary works, section by section. Each page represents one day of activity.

Start by writing in the date, time, and location of your workout (gym, home, yoga studio, outdoors, etc.) at the top of each page.

Date: _____ Time: _____
Location: ☐ Gym ☐ Home ☐ Other: _____

In the next section, "Overall Sequence," you'll provide a *summary* of your workout: a snapshot of that day's routine, intensity, and results. (*Lower down we'll note details about each exercise in the sequence.*)

OVERALL SEQUENCE
Rate intensity from 1 (lowest) to 10 (highest)
1. Exercise Type: _____ Duration: _____ Intensity: _____ Response: A _____ O _____

- For type of exercise, fill in what you did, such as: biking, treadmill, etc.

- For duration, fill in the length of time spent on this activity.

- For exertion intensity, on a scale of 1 to 10—with 1 being low and 10 being high—rate your level of exertion.

- For response, after the "A" for arousal, fill in "yes" or "no" if you experienced arousal; after the "O" for orgasm, fill in "yes" or "no" if you reached orgasm.

For example, let's say you biked for 30 minutes at a moderate intensity and didn't experience any arousal or orgasm. That section would look like this:

1. Exercise Type: ___bike___ Duration: _30 mins._ Intensity: _5_ Response: A _no_ O _no_

For a different scenario, if you did a pretty intense elliptical workout for 45 minutes and then did an ab workout at a high intensity for 10 minutes, and experienced arousal during the ab workout, then your sequence information might look like the following:

1. Exercise Type: _elliptical_ Duration: _45 mins._ Intensity: _8_ Response: A _no_ O _no_
2. Exercise Type: _ab workout_ Duration: _10 mins._ Intensity: _9_ Response: A _yes_ O _no_

Next, you'll want to document information about your cardio workout, if you did any.

CARDIO

1. Indicate whether you did your cardio before ab work, after ab work, or N/A if you didn't do any cardio at all. If you did cardio before abs, note how many minutes passed between finishing your cardio and starting your abs. Also note the length of the cardio workout.

2. Indicate the exercise you did (running, biking, etc.). If it's not listed, write what you did after "Other."

3. Indicate the intensity of your cardio workout (using a scale from 1 to 10). If it wasn't at all intense (e.g., if your heart rate felt relaxed and you could have easily carried on a conversation for ages), then you'd rate it as 1. More moderately intense workouts would be somewhere in the middle, like 4, 5, or 6. And if you're breathing really hard and finding it a little more difficult to carry on a conversation, you might rate it 7. If the intensity is ramped up and you're giving it all you've got—and couldn't possibly carry on a conversation—you're probably working out in the 8–10 range.

4. Next, document your level of arousal using a scale from 1 to 10, with 1 being not at all aroused and 10 being very aroused (a 9 or 10 would be so aroused you're feeling close to orgasm).

5. If you experienced arousal or orgasm, note the point in time during the workout at which it occurred.

If you ran for 30 minutes at a level 7 of intensity and started feeling moderately aroused (level 5) after about 20 minutes of running, this section would look like the following:

Cardio: ☐ Before Abs ☐ After Abs ☐ N/A
If Cardio Before Abs, how much time passed between cardio and abs? _____ mins
Cardio length: __30_ mins
☒ Running ☐ Elliptical ☐ Biking ☐ Stairmaster ☐ Other _____
Cardio intensity? (1 to 10; 1=not at all; 10=very): __7_
A (1 to 10; 1=not at all; 10=very): __5_ O: ☐ Yes ☐ No ☐ Close
If A, when: at _20_ min
If O, when: at _____ min

For each section marked "Exercise 1" or "Exercise 2" (and so on), there is space to write the kind of exercise you did, such as leg lifts, squats, bicep curls, crunches, or planks. This section is perfect for keeping tracking of strength training and ab exercises.

By now you are probably getting the hang of this. Here's what you do:

1. **EXERCISE:** Write in the kind of exercise you did (e.g., crunches, leg raises, jack-knives, bicep curls, etc.).

2. **REPS:** Document how many reps you did (and whether you did all those reps in a row, without stopping; or whether you did them in sets, such as two sets of 10).

3. **RESULT:** If you experienced arousal, note the level. For orgasm, indicate "yes," "no," or "close." If neither, leave it blank.

4. **TIMING:** A. if you started feeling aroused, note after how many reps it began. Do the same for orgasm. B. If you were lifting weights, indicate how many pounds the weights were and whether this was light, medium, or difficult for you.

Thus, if you did 60 crunches in three sets of 20, had very strong arousal (level 9) beginning after about 35 crunches, and you felt close to an orgasm, then your diary would look like the section below (notice the weight section is blank because you didn't lift any weights):

EXERCISE 1: _____ crunches _____
\# Reps: _60_ (____ all at once? Or _3_ sets of _20_)
A (1 to 10; 1 = not at all; 10 = very): _9_
O: ☐ Yes ☐ No ☒ Close
At what rep did A start? _35_ At what rep O? _____
If weights: ____ lbs; ☐ light for you ☐ medium ☐ difficult

Notes

As you recall, the "C" in C.O.R.E. stands for challenging yourself. That's why this diary shows whether you were challenging yourself, and to what degree, from day to day. Choosing a number for the intensity also has a way of making that effort more tangible, which could inspire you to push for a 7 tomorrow if you gave a 5 today. The diary also helps you see what patterns are true for you, since every woman is a little different. While some women may feel aroused after doing 30 or 40 crunches, that might do little to nothing for you. You might find that you start feeling aroused in the middle of your second set of leg raises or during an intense set of planks. Try to be open to your experience. The Coregasm Workout provides the tools and the methods, but it's up to you to put it into practice!

The diary template accommodates up to ten different exercises for one day, which has been more than enough for most of the women in our research. If you need more space, you can always start a second sheet; or, keep track of just the exercises you feel are important for understanding your patterns of arousal.

Remember: order matters. Keeping a diary can help you figure out what order of exercise works for you. That information can help you develop a few routines that are both fun and challenging, and that just might help you connect more deeply with your body.

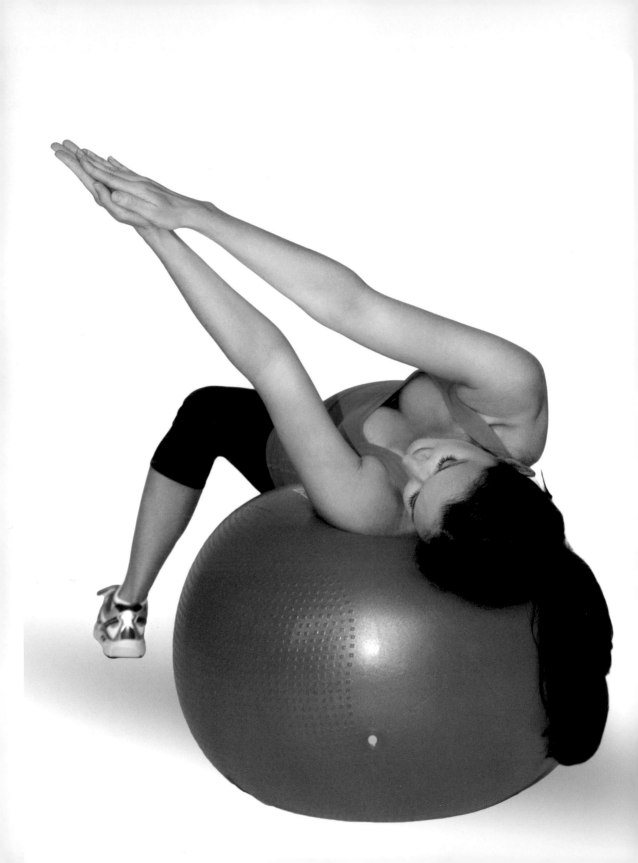

Some of the women in our research who started having exercise-induced arousal wondered, *Were the arousal feelings always there and I just never noticed them before?*

It's a good question. Too often, we women feel closed off from our bodies—and for any number of reasons. Some women have internalized the taunts they got in school about being too fat or too skinny or too tall or too short. Some women experience unwanted attention directed at their butt or their breasts, and as a result "cover up" to avoid harassment on the street. Other women feel disconnected because of past sexual abuse or sexual assault, which all too many women around the world can relate to. (If you're healing from sexual abuse or assault, consider meeting with a counselor or therapist. See the appendix for resources.) If any of the above sounds familiar to you, it's possible you've tried to disconnect from your body—consciously or unconsciously. Many of us probably do that at some time or another. Unfortunately, extended disconnection prevents us from tapping into the natural feelings of sensuality and sexuality we all have a right to. That's what I hope the Coregasm Workout can do for you: help you connect with your body and its sensations so you can notice your body's natural inclinations toward arousal and desire.

With that in mind, when you exercise try to notice how you feel all over. Do you feel warm? Sweaty? When do you start to sweat? Which exercises feel playful or fun to you? Which exercises feel exciting to you in a challenging way? Are there others you just don't like? Which exercises make your heart pound or your muscles quiver? Try to pay attention to how your body feels so you can include more of the exercises you like and fewer of those you don't. This is *your* workout—you should have fun doing it! And try to notice when you feel warm or breathy, when your heart pounds, or when you feel happy or aroused. Answers to any and all of these questions indicate an increasing awareness of your body, listening to what it has to tell you. You can transfer this awareness to sex, too, noticing exactly how you feel with your partner. How do you feel when your partner kisses you, let's say, on your ear? What about on your neck? Or your inner thighs? When you become more aware of what kinds of touch turn you on, or what kinds of talk—from dirty to romantic to silence—you like, you'll be able to fine-tune the sex life that feels best to you, and partly by also sharing those turn-ons and turn-offs with your partner, providing a road map to your pleasure.

5 [It would start] really low inside, like inside the genital area . . . rather than just necessarily outside stimulation. After yoga, especially during meditation, just being really relaxed, like after doing some [yoga] positions and being really slow and fluid about it and then just relaxing and meditating and sitting in the lotus position and just relaxing, yeah, a wave would just come over me.

—ELIZABETH

CHAPTER 5

C.O.R.E. PRINCIPLE 3:
RELAX AND RECEIVE

MANY WOMEN SEEK assistance in hopes of increasing sexual desire, satisfaction, or arousal. In recent years, a variety of pharmaceutical medications have been used in clinical trials to treat women's sexual difficulties. Many of these have been used in hopes of increasing women's sexual desire, satisfaction, or arousal. Yet, so far, most medications tested have been shown to be pretty ineffective for these sexual concerns.

These disappointing results led doctors and scientists to explore alternative approaches to treating sexual difficulties, including healthy lifestyle changes like exercise as well as Eastern philosophies and practices like mindfulness, tantra, and yoga, which have a history thousands of years in the making. Those who came generations before us understood how to tap into the wisdom of our bodies and minds; their teachings spoke to the importance of relaxing, of allowing oneself to receive.

Many people in our studies described how exercise arousal and orgasm helped them adopt a mindset of receptivity. They chose to open themselves to their mind-body experience and follow where those feelings led them.

Now, this might sound contradictory to what you've been reading so far, especially after so many people's accounts of reaching successful arousal through strenuous exercise. Though many have described exercising with intensity, their intensity isn't

Smoking and nicotine have long been linked to sexual difficulties, including erectile problems for men and arousal difficulties for women. In fact, in some countries you can find advertisements that depict a sagging cigarette where a man's penis would be. Not very sexy, is it?

The good news is that studies have shown that sexual function can improve after a person quits smoking. If you smoke, it might be time to consider really working to conquer this difficult habit. Fortunately, once you do decide, there are medical professionals and helpful smoking cessation programs just waiting to assist you. Your loved ones will thank you, as will your heart, lungs, and pocketbook.

necessarily frenzied; it's *focused*. Being "in the zone" while running, swimming, or pedaling can feel relaxing without feeling stressful.

The emphasis of this book on increasing intensity and challenge in your workouts still stands—it just does so alongside another finding. Our research reveals that being present and open to your experiences is also important—whether during exercise or when exploring your own sexuality. And so this is the *R* in C.O.R.E.—relaxing into and receiving the feelings your body experiences, knowing that exercise, like sex, can be fun, playful, and exploratory.

RECEIVING COREGASM

Throughout our research, participants have described in pretty standard phrasing how they "reached" or "achieved" orgasm. But in our conversations with Mary, whom we met in earlier chapters, I noticed she always spoke in terms of "receiving the coregasm," as if her exercise orgasm was a gift that just happened to her. For example: "When I'm at the gym, at the very end, and I'm doing my ab workout, that's when I usually just let it happen because I know my body is so exhausted I'm going to receive a coregasm." She also described sex orgasms as something she and her partner received. However they happened, Mary consistently had a positive, playful attitude about orgasm.

Curious about her perspective, I asked her to say more. Mary's idea was this: although she had to physically challenge herself in order to fatigue her muscles, once she reached that point she could simply relax into and receive the coregasm, which she saw as her reward at the end of her workout. She explained: "During sex it takes a while for your body to reach orgasm, and I feel like it's very similar for coregasms as well. It takes your body some time to warm up and get the muscles moving."

This idea of "receiving" coregasm stayed with me, particularly as we kept interviewing woman after woman who talked about feeling particularly relaxed when experiencing orgasm during exercise. Some described zoning out, such as Lyla, who regularly experienced orgasms while running on the treadmill or using the elliptical. She'd listen to music with strong bass beats and would concentrate on the music, and the next thing she knew, she'd be sweating, running faster, and in the midst of a coregasm. This mental component, this "zoning out," this concentration and focus, was apparent with many of the women we spoke with. They didn't just facilitate the physical intensity of the exercise; they also allowed themselves to connect, to feel at one with their music or their body, and to be open to whatever bodily sensations came their way.

Ultimately, this is an example of what's called the mind-body connection, which plays as much a role in exercise as it does in sex. Your mind and your thoughts either work with you—encouraging you to keep going, reminding you that you're powerful and sexy and lovable—or they work against you—telling you to quit or give up, that you're not worth it. Your mind has such a powerful influence on sex that sex educators commonly cite how "the brain is the biggest sex organ." For one thing, the brain activates certain kinds of arousal and orgasm. But our brains also control how we feel about ourselves as people, how we feel about our bodies, and what we know or don't know about sex. Our brains house all the pleasant, painful, scary, exciting, and arousing memories and feelings about sex from our pasts—and all those old thoughts and feelings influence our sex lives in the present.

Fortunately, we can invite, even train, our minds to work with us rather than against us, and exercise is an excellent means of doing this. Becoming more mindful of and present to what our bodies feel as we exercise can help us more easily receive exercise-induced arousal and orgasm. But even if you don't experience such arousal, or if you don't particularly seek it, becoming more mindful of and present to what our bodies feel at the gym can only help us feel more mindful and present in the bedroom.

To follow are some common and effective ways to open ourselves to our bodily sensations.

THE PRACTICE OF YOGA

Numerous recent studies have demonstrated the many benefits of practicing the ancient tradition of yoga, including improving the sexual response.

Practicing yoga has been shown to benefit our physical health in a number of ways, such as reducing stress, improving sleep, lifting depression, lowering blood pressure, and even expanding lung capacity.

Yoga seems to benefit our emotional, even spiritual, health as well. Yoga has been shown to help with attention and breathing and with developing more positive feelings, greater body awareness, and a generally greater satisfaction with life. Those who practice yoga may also find they feel less stressed or anxious—relaxed conditions that likely set the stage for easier arousal and more pleasurable sex.

Research also suggests that some yoga practices may improve certain sexual responses: premature ejaculation and ejaculatory control in men, and sexual desire, lubrication, and arousal in women. One study in particular found that practicing yoga twice a week for three months improved blood pressure, sexual arousal, vaginal lubrication, and overall sexual function among Korean women with metabolic syndrome. The hour-long yoga classes of the study, like many yoga classes, focused on about fourteen yoga poses (*asanas*) plus focused breathing (*pranayama*). These classes would always end with relaxation through the corpse pose (*shavasana*).

Of course, none of this yoga research studied the potential of yoga to cause arousal or orgasm. And yet, starting in 2011, various websites published articles about so-called yogasms, many of which sounded like the exercise-induced orgasms that involve relaxation. In our research, quite a few women reported it was yoga that induced their exercise arousal. Some women, like Elizabeth and Christina, felt it was the mindful, meditative state they experienced that facilitated their orgasms. Researchers are just beginning to explore the possible overlap between orgasm and mindful or meditative states of consciousness, such as how the brain's prefrontal cortex becomes active during some meditative states in the same manner as it does during certain types of female orgasm— particularly for women who can experience orgasm through thought alone.

Other women in our studies believed it was certain ways of stretching or moving muscles in yoga that triggered their arousal, such as with the pigeon pose or standing- or seated-forward bends. Louann shared:

I have no idea why, but doing Bikram yoga really does it. Specific postures include: Hands to Feet, Standing Separate Leg Stretching, Standing Separate Leg Head to Knee, Dead Body [corpse pose], Wind Removing, sit-ups, Locust, Half Tortoise, and Sitting Head to Knee. I was really surprised—pleasantly surprised—at my body's response.

Some women felt that any exercise resembling sexual positions—some common, like the cow (like rear entry/doggie-style) or bridge (like some versions of missionary); some not so common, like the plough (legs up and over one's head)—could lead to arousal. One told us that holding the yoga positions that mimic sexual positions, combined with deep breathing, relaxation, and a heightened mind-body connection, forged her sexual arousal.

All of this is to say that, regardless of any sexual arousal or orgasm you may experience from practicing yoga, there are myriad reasons to give it a try—physical, emotional, spiritual, and sensual.

To follow you'll find several core exercises that utilize yoga poses: tree pose, downward-facing dog, three-legged dog, pigeon pose, and lotus lift.

TREE

Tree pose is a lovely part of many yoga classes, as it adds a sense of calm and centering to the practice. It's also a great way to learn and practice balance.

1. Stand with your feet facing forward about hip-width apart.

2. Slowly lift one foot up and press it against the side of your opposite calf or your inner thigh. Do not press it against your knee!

3. Move your hands into a prayer-like pose either in front of your chest or above your head (*as pictured*). (Ideally you'd lift your foot and hands into position simultaneously.)

4. Slowly breathe in and out. Initially try to hold this pose for 3–5 full breaths. As you improve your balance, try to hold the pose for at least 10 complete slow breaths.

5. When you're ready, slowly lower your leg and arms back down. Shake your body a bit to loosen up.

6. Repeat on the opposite side.

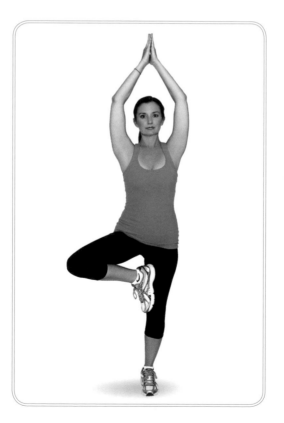

DOWNWARD-FACING DOG

Downward-facing dog (also called downward dog) is another yoga favorite that's a great stretch at the start or end of a workout. It can also provide moments of calm in the midst of an intense practice.

1. Stand with your feet planted shoulder-width apart. (See also variant tip, below.)

2. Hinge forward from your hips, planting your hands palm-down on the ground shoulder-width apart. (It's okay if your heels don't touch the floor.)

3. Make sure that your head and back form a straight line (*as pictured*). Keeping this straight line, try to lengthen your back, pushing your hips into the air. Hold this pose for several breaths.

Tips

- You can also start on your hands and knees. Next you'd push up to the ceiling and straighten your knees or, keeping your knees slightly bent, you could try to lower your heels toward the floor.

Ways to Challenge Yourself

- Since people vary in their flexibility, you may find your heels don't touch the floor and never will; that's okay. As you practice, just gently try to lower your heels as much as you can.

- As you become more comfortable and flexible in this pose, you may find yourself able to sink lower into it so that your head is in line with your arms. Just be sure to keep your head and back in a straight line.

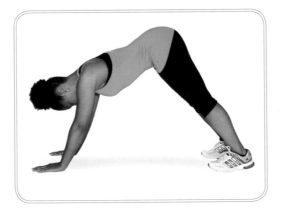

THREE-LEGGED DOG

A variation on downward-facing dog is the three-legged dog, in which you simply lift one leg and hold it in the air (*as pictured*) for several breaths. Then switch sides.

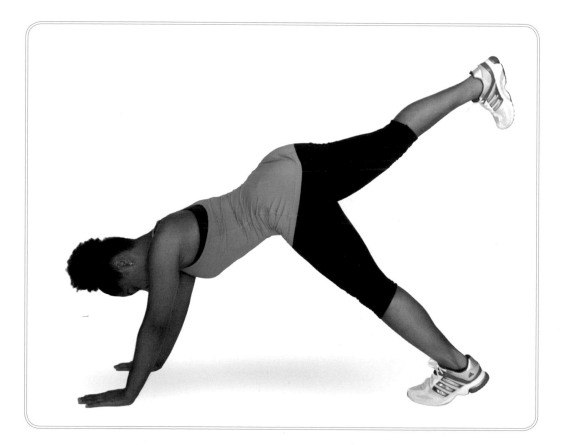

PIGEON

Pigeon is a challenging pose that requires some flexibility in the hips and glutes. If you're not there yet, don't worry; you'll get more flexible with practice. (If you have any knee concerns, work with a personal trainer at first, or skip this exercise.)

1. Start on your hands and knees in a tabletop position, with your hands in line with your shoulders and your knees in line with your hips.

2. Bring your right knee toward your chest and then through your arms. Your right thigh and knee should now be in front of your right hip socket. Be careful not to let your knee slidet out to the right; it should stay in front of your body.

3. At the same time, stretch your left leg to the back so that it's in a straight line, with the instep (top) of your foot touching the floor.

4. With your hands still planted on the floor and your chest open, make sure you're facing forward (*pictured, left*). Breathe in and out for 5–10 slow and easy breaths if you're able. This is a perfectly good stopping point.

5. If you want to take the pose farther into full pigeon, fold forward (*pictured, right*), rounding over your front leg and folding your arms on the floor. Breathe in and out, holding the pose for 5–10 breaths if you can.

6. When you're ready, lift up your arms and head, then bring your legs back to a tabletop or seated position. Shake your body out a little.

7. Repeat on the other side.

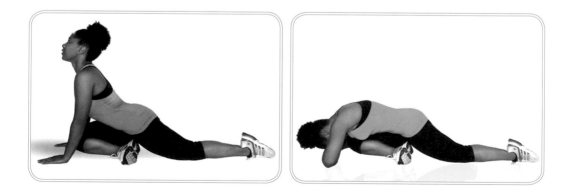

LOTUS LIFT

The lotus lift is not for everyone; it can be pretty tricky given the flexibility and strength it requires. It's easier if you can first get into a lotus position, with each foot over the opposite thigh (easier when barefoot).

1. Start in lotus position with each foot resting on the opposite thigh (*pictured, left*). Hinge forward slightly at the hips.

2. Place your hands, palms down, on the floor on either side of your hip bones. Your hands should be underneath your shoulders.

3. Try pushing into the ground through the palms of your hands while lifting your seated body upward (*pictured, right*). (I find this easier to do if I first tilt my knees upward and closer to my torso.) The result is that your hips come off the ground, leaving your body supported entirely by your hands.

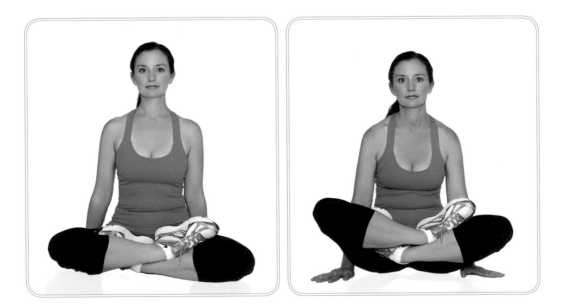

COREGASM 101 WHAT'S YOUR MANTRA?

Some practitioners of yoga include mantras in their practice—Sanskrit words, such as *om* used to focus the mind—or *kriyas*, which may combine mantras, breath, and postures. And some of the men from our research shared that using *kriyas* helped them experience orgasm, whether as part of exercise or part of sex.

But you don't have to be seriously into yoga or tantra to learn how to relax and receive, just as you don't need to be an expert meditator in order to live more mindfully. You can actually meditate, relax, and receive simultaneously just by focusing on your breath: breathing in, breathing out. You might also think *Breathe in* as you slowly inhale, and then *Breathe out* as you slowly exhale. Some count as they breathe: four counts for the inhale, six for the exhale. (Since that's ten seconds, if you counted for six breaths, focusing on each inhale and exhale, you would have successfully meditated for one full minute.)

Any practice simply takes practice. And reassurance. To provide that reassurance, some people repeat to themselves encouraging phrases, such as *You can do this*. And you know what? You *can* do this. You can commit to exercise. You can open yourself to your sensuality and your sexuality. You can do it all.

MINDFUL ATTENTION

Cultivating mindfulness isn't just about taking the time to smell the roses; it's about actually savoring each rose that you smell.

Stop for a moment and consider: How often do you engage in an activity while simultaneously thinking about something else? Perhaps you stress over your to-do list while sitting in class or driving the kids to school. Or during your workout you ruminate over that awkward conversation with your boss. Or how about when you're having sex: Have your thoughts ever strayed to that upcoming work presentation or to whether you unplugged the iron?

Mindfulness is the practice of being in the present moment. In other words, fully experiencing whatever we're currently doing: tasting our food, enjoying our swim, listening to our kids, gratefully relaxing under the covers at the end of the day. But practicing mindfulness is more than just deciding to notice the roses; it's an ongoing process with numerous benefits. For one, mindfulness training can help us reduce stress. A mind that's focused on the here and now is—in that moment—a mind that's neither dwelling on the past nor worrying about the future. Mindfulness helps us experience life right in the moment, whether we're breathing in the scent of morning air or feeling "in the zone" on an intense run.

Many women in our exercise diary study said that tracking their sexual responses to exercise made them feel more connected to and aware of their bodily sensations. They said learning to experience arousal made them more motivated to exercise or to challenge themselves during exercise. And when you're more aware of your bodily sensations in relation to exercise, you're likely to be more aware of your bodily sensations in relation to sex and romance.

Indeed, University of British Columbia psychologist Lori Brotto found that women engaged in mindfulness-based therapies became more aware of their physical sensations related to sexual arousal, and with this awareness they could open themselves to feeling more sexually aroused. This is valuable information, for other studies have shown that women are particularly prone to what we scientists call "cognitive distractions" during sex—thinking about anything other than the sex we're engaging in. And even when we are aware of our sexual engagement, too often we're focused on how our thighs or breasts or stomach look rather than on what we're experiencing with our partner. (Men have these self-conscious distracting thoughts too, especially regarding their sexual performance.)

Mindfulness training has helped many women improve their sexual desire and arousal. When people feel more in tune with their bodies, they're more likely to notice warmth, tingling, or increased lubrication. Noticing these physiological signals of arousal can lead to psychological arousal. And once arousal enters conscious awareness, it's easier to relax into the experience and receive pleasure. Whether you're making love or eating chocolate or stretching your quads, being present allows you to connect with your body in the moment.

So how do we train in mindfulness? Essentially, we "tone" it like a muscle: starting small, practicing regularly, and increasing over time. Exercise can provide an excellent space for practicing mindfulness, one where we can work to focus without judgment on every stride, stretch, stroke, kick, or rep. Below I describe how to walk mindfully, but let's start with something everyone does every day.

Eating Mindfully

So many of us eat mindlessly. We regularly bite, chew, and swallow without truly noticing taste and aroma and texture—let alone considering what we're putting into our bodies, or how it will benefit us, or where it came from and how it reached our plates. Try to slow the process of taking in nourishment; try to savor each nibble, relish each sip.

1. Start with a small morsel of food: a raisin, a grape, an olive, a raspberry.

2. Consider what it is, where it came from. An Italian hillside? A California orchard? A local farm? Consider the route it likely took to reach you, as well as all the people who were a part of that process.

3. Look at it. Study its surface: wrinkled or smooth, shiny or dull. Notice its color: vibrant red, deep purple, dusky green.

4. Sniff it. How would you describe its scent?

5. Place it in your mouth. Pay attention to how it feels on your tongue, against your cheek, on the roof of your mouth.

6. Roll it with your tongue; chew it with your teeth. Notice its flavor, its texture, its flesh, its juice.

7. Swallow this morsel only after you've kept it in your mouth for at least 10–20 seconds.

A great reason to start mindfulness training with eating is that most of us *love* food and love eating it. And yet that fact doesn't stop us from consuming our meals on autopilot. As long as we've gone so far as to purchase and/or prepare the delectibles before us, why not glean as much benefit and appreciation as we can out of them? The more we can cultivate our awareness in specific activities, the more we'll be able to enjoy and appreciate all our activities.

Walking Mindfully

Now, let's consider how we can more mindfully engage in another daily practice: the act of regularly putting one foot in front of the other. Try it first barefoot, in a small space; then take this method out into the big world, wherever you happen to be, wherever you happen to be going.

INDOORS

1. Take one step as slowly as you can. Take another. Focus on how your feet feel with each step, the gentle rolling sensation from the heel to the toes. Pay attention to the floor beneath your feet. Is it soft carpet? Smooth hardwood? Slick tile? Spongy matting? Textured concrete? Notice the sensations in your foot as you press it against the floor, how the other foot feels as you lift it to join its mate. Consider how your body balances itself between your feet, both forward to back and side to side. Feel your hands hanging at your sides, how gently your fingertips brush against your thighs.

2. When you feel you've thoroughly contemplated walking indoors, put on shoes.

OUTDOORS

3. Now, head out the door to take a stroll. First maintain your attention on your feet, noting the sensations of each step. Note the surface you walk on, be it brick, concrete, grass, asphalt, gravel, bark, or dirt.

4. Next consider other physical sensations: the warmth of the sun, the caress of the breeze.

5. Bring in other senses. What do you see? Identify the colors of the objects you see, the variations in shape and design. A striped shirt? A sparkling sidewalk? Variegated leaves? Are those leaves falling? Are there kids running?

6. What do you smell: Grass and dirt, herbs and flowers? Car exhaust and hot sidewalk? Aromas wafting from the bakery you just passed, or the coffee roastery? The oregano of pizza sauce or the clay of an art class?

7. What sounds come to your attention: Birds twittering? Car engines rumbling? The rustle of leaves? Bells or sirens or whistles? Conversation and the steps of passersby?

8. Notice anything and everything. Notice and name your passing thoughts and sensations: "I feel the wind blowing." "I see leaves falling." "I hear streetcars rumbling." Notice and acknowledge and name and experience—and let each item fall away.

Now, of course most of us don't have the freedom to walk mindfully everywhere we go. But ideally, you'll be able to take a mindful walk somewhat regularly, even just for short periods of time. As you continue practicing, you'll likely find it's easier to notice and appreciate the world around you—even when you're rushing to a meeting or scrambling to get home in time for dinner. As you become practiced in mindfulness, you'll find that these places of peace and attention are yours for the noticing any time you need them.

Mindful Exercise

Now, let's see if we can apply some of these same moments of conscious attention to how we exercise—whatever that exercise may be.

1. First, notice your breath. Try to keep breathing steadily no matter what you're doing. Is your breath quickening? Slow and deep? What does it feel like to close your eyes as you breathe in and out, even if for just a moment?

2. Next, notice your heart and heart rate. Is it pounding, the blood coursing through your veins? Does your heart rate feel calm and steady as you hold a stretch?

3. Consider the sensations on your skin. Perhaps you feel the sweat and hot air of a heated yoga class? The breeze as you zip along on your bike? The smooth, caressing water supporting your breaststroke?

4. Consider, too, your muscles and joints, the energy flowing throughout your body, and the alternating tension and relaxation of working your reps.

It's conscious attention that helps us get more in tune with the rhythms of our bodies.

Mindful Massage

Massage takes touch to the level of connecting with a partner. This is best done when wearing as few clothes as possible. Also, using a massage lotion or oil allows your hands to glide more easily over your partner's body.

1. Have your partner lie facedown on a bed.

2. Begin by slowly moving your hands up and down your partner's back.

3. At times, keep your hands still, gently pressing your hands on your partner's back and feeling the warmth of his or her skin.

4. Experiment with your technique: at times use your whole hand, at times just a single finger, just the palm, just the fingertips.

5. As you touch your partner, notice how the touch feels physically. But also try to notice how you feel emotionally. Do you feel love? Arousal? Contentment? Sadness or happiness? Nostalgia? Pay attention to all your thoughts and feelings; this is a process of connecting your physical and emotional experiences into one enriched experience.

6. Try to spend at least 3 to 5 minutes on your partner's back before switching roles.

With time and practice, we can all become more present-minded—which will enable us to better enjoy all the moments we have.

There's a reason exercise is described as mind-body experience. The mind plays an important role in how we feel about our bodies, as well as in how much we notice our bodily sensations. Regardless of whether you choose to explore relaxation or mindfulness or work on openness so that you can feel more comfortable receiving these or other feelings, I hope you enjoy the journey.

I find it pleasurable to fantasize while riding my bike or hiking. I think the slight touch of my thighs, along with my enjoyment of the outdoors, makes it easy to feel sexy and good about myself.

—LISETTE

Because of my coregasm experiences, I was able to really learn about my body—the way it works, what exercises can trigger it, how fast it will take me. And so when I started having more consistent sex I was able to work my body and kind of push myself and tense my muscles to receive a stronger or faster orgasm. And it's been great because my partner and I are able to, most of the time, receive orgasm at the same time. When I sense he's on the verge I can purposely really tense my muscles hard and receive an orgasm. He asks: "Was it me, or was it your coregasm?" It's probably a little bit of both; me tensing my muscles, and him.

—MARY

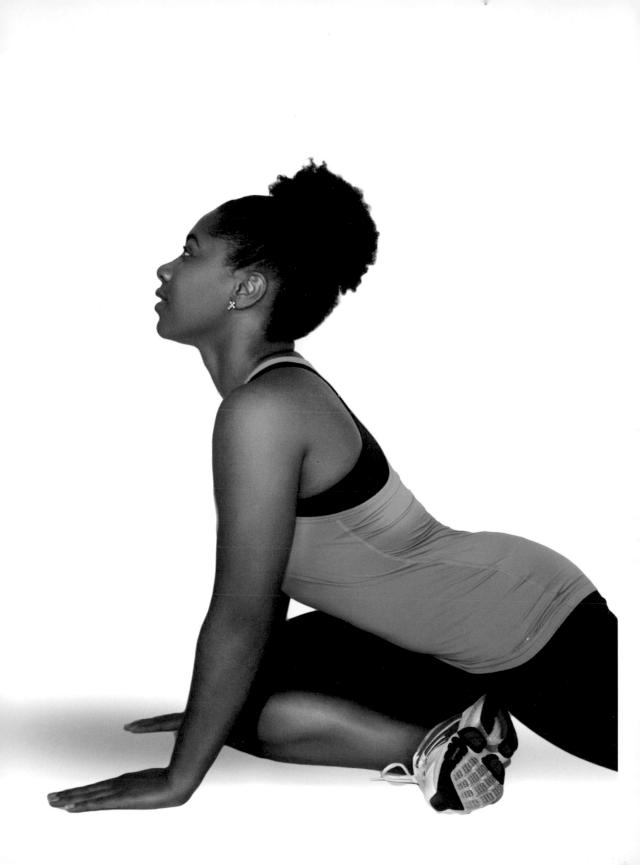

6 The sexual pleasure I have nearly always accompanies some kind of abdomen strain. Sit-ups when I am really working out my lower abdominal muscles. When I was mopping the store I worked at as a teenager, the bearing-down sensation was felt in my lower abdomen—almost like a warming, tingling sensation with pressure in my pelvic region. I need this same kind of pressure in order to orgasm when I'm having sex (either solo or partnered) by tilting or thrusting my hips.

—VERA

CHAPTER 6

C.O.R.E. PRINCIPLE 4: ENGAGE YOUR LOWER ABS

THE *E* IN C.O.R.E. stands for "Engage"— and specifically, "Engage your lower abs." That doesn't mean that the lower abs are the only ones working. As noted earlier, it's common for ab exercises to engage a number of core muscles at the same time, including muscles in and around the abs, back, and hips. That ab exercises tend to involve several muscles is good for our bodies, because it means individual exercises can train multiple muscles. But that fact has also made it difficult to unravel some of the more mysterious parts of how exactly coregasms work. This is true for sex, too.

Take the G-spot as an example. After all, there's a lot packed closely together in the genital area (e.g., the urethra, vagina, spongy tissues, nerves, etc.) and so, for women who respond to G-spot stimulation it's unclear why it feels erotic and even orgasmic to so many women. Is it the nerves in the front wall of the vagina? Erectile tissue around the urethra? The inside branches of the clitoris (called the crura)? All of the above? Coregasms present a similar mystery.

CORE EXERCISE BASICS

To follow are some basics about core exercise to prime you for the Coregasm Workout. And again, please consult with your doctor or physical therapist before beginning any new exercise regimen; health experts can provide essential information on how to tailor any workout to suit your particular pain, injury, or medical risks or concerns. (For example, if you're prone to low back pain, you may want to skip crunches, which move the spine, and instead do planks, which strengthen stability.)

First, warm up by walking for a few minutes.

When you begin the Coregasm Workout, perhaps after some cardio work, **ease into the first few minutes with cat/cow and bridge.** Next, head into planks—prone, supine, or side.

Core exercises can involve movement (such as with crunches) **or can be static** (such as plank), in which we stiffen the core muscles. You'll find both types in the Coregasm Workout.

It's important to vary your workout from time to time. Remember: since so many different muscles make up the core, no single exercise can adequately engage or challenge every core muscle. And since we all have different fitness goals, no single core exercise routine will suit everyone. Choose from the various exercises in the Coregasm Workout, and mix them up. Even if you find some favorites, be sure to include a healthy range of exercises in your routine.

Be sure to include some functional exercises in your routine. Functional exercises train your muscles to successfully work together for everyday movements like getting up from a chair, lifting a toddler into a car seat, and putting away groceries. Take squats: regularly practicing squats can help ensure that, as we age, we can still sit down and get up again safely. Or picture yourself sitting on the floor with an infant, scooping her up, and then cradling her back and forth; in a workout, similar movements might include a Russian twist with a medicine ball. And medicine ball slams can be practice for playing games like box ball or basketball with kids. Functional exercises apply to sex, too. As you continue practicing various exercises in the Coregasm Workout—especially cat/cow, bridge, prone plank, supine plank, crunches, and downward-facing dog —you'll be primed for having fun with similar sexual positions for decades to come.

COREGASM 101 RISE AND SHINE BEFORE WORKING THE SPINE

Experts in spine health recommend waiting to do spinal exercises—including the lower abdominal exercises of this chapter—until after you've been awake for at least an hour. Why? There is greater pressure on the disks shortly after you awaken, which means there is greater risk of injury. So, if you're a morning exerciser, you'd be wise to avoid these movements for at least one hour, after which your body should be better situated for core exercises.

Take it slowly and be patient with yourself. The core is an essential part of your being, and it should be treated with care. So go slowly, both at the start and each time you progress. That means, as you experiment with Coregasm Workout exercises, try just a few reps at first to see how your body responds. Or if it's an exercise you hold for a period of time, at first just hold it for 10 seconds; if that goes well, hold for longer next time. If something doesn't feel right, listen to your body, and discontinue the exercise until you can discuss it with your physical therapist, doctor, or personal trainer.

SIDE PLANK

The side plank is a common variation of the prone plank. It engages both the lower abdominal muscles and the obliques.

1. Lie on your left side with your legs together, the upper leg resting on the lower leg. With your left arm bent, and using your elbow and forearm for support, prop up your torso (*pictured, left*). Your elbow should be directly under your shoulder.

2. Squeeze your core as you lift your hips and extend your right arm toward the ceiling (*pictured, right*). Your legs and hips should be lifted above the floor; only your feet, elbow, and forearm should be touching the floor.

3. Make sure your body is in a straight line from your ankles to your shoulders.

4. Breathe in and out and try to hold the pose for 10 seconds.

5. Repeat on the other side.

Ways to Challenge Yourself

- Work up to holding the plank for 30–60 seconds. Some people even strive for holding planks for several minutes!

- You can also try any variation on lifting your top leg 6 inches or higher and holding it for 30 seconds or longer.

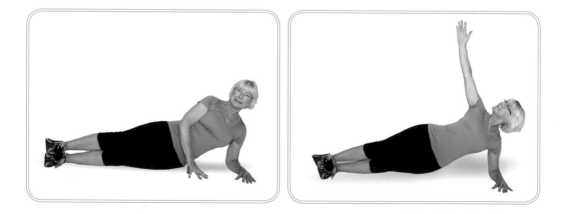

SUPINE PLANK

Supine ("soo-pine") simply means that your front is facing upward. The supine plank works the posterior (back) muscles, such as the glutes, hamstrings, and lower back.

1. Sit on the floor with your hands, palms down, behind you (*pictured, left*).

2. Keeping your core squeezed and tight, simultaneously lift your hips off the floor while pressing your hands against the floor (*pictured, right*). Only your heels and palms should be touching the floor, with your toes pointing straight up.

3. Make sure your body forms a straight line from your head to your ankles.

4. Breathe in and out. Try to hold the pose for at least 10 seconds.

Ways to Challenge Yourself

- Work up to holding the pose for 30–60 seconds. When you're ready, try to hold it for 1–2 minutes.

- You can also try lifting one leg slightly off the ground.

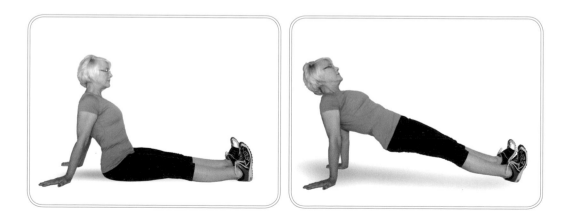

CRUNCHES

Crunches are a common core exercise that most of us can do, regardless of our fitness level. They can induce arousal in some people.

1. Lie flat on your back with your knees bent and your feet flat on the floor, hip-width apart.

2. Place your hands behind your head, with your thumbs behind your ears (*pictured, top*). Keep your hands apart; do not lace your fingers together.

3. To crunch straight up, squeeze your core abdominal muscles (making them super stiff) and lift your shoulders and chest a few inches off the floor with your head lifted toward the ceiling. Hold this for a moment and then slowly lower down.

4. To crunch to the right side, squeeze your abs while lifting your left shoulder just a few inches off the floor toward your right side (*pictured, bottom*).

5. To crunch to the left side, squeeze your abs while lifting your right shoulder just a few inches off the floor toward your left side. Alternate between crunching straight up and to the left and right. Aim for 10 crunches in each direction (30 total).

Tips

- Do not pull on your neck and do not push your head with your hands; your abs should be doing the work here.

- If you have lower back pain or a back injury, skip crunches until you have a chance to talk with your doctor, physical therapist, or personal trainer to see if they are okay for you.

- Try to maintain a slow, controlled movement.

Ways to Challenge Yourself

- Do crunches to the point of fatigue; just be sure to keep good form.

- You can also lift your feet in the air (at roughly a 90-degree angle) by either propping them on a chair or by holding them as if they were resting on a chair.

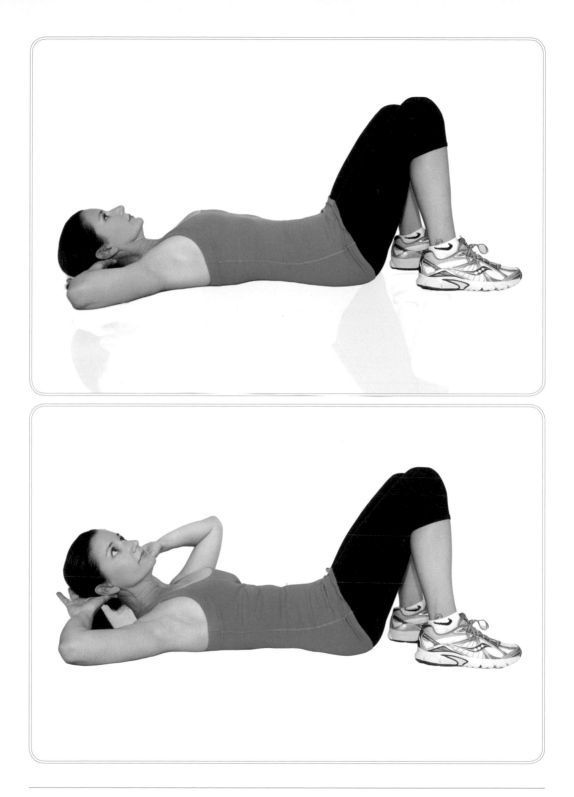

EXTENDED BICYCLE CRUNCH

The extended bicycle crunch is similar to a regular bicycle crunch, except both legs remain straight.

1. Lie on your back with your legs straight up at a 90-degree angle to the floor. Your hands should be behind your head, but don't interlace your fingers (*pictured, left*).

2. Crunch to the right: keeping your right leg straight in the air, simultaneously lower your left leg toward the floor while drawing your elbow toward the opposite leg (*pictured, right*). If you are new to extended bicycle crunches, it's okay to lower your left leg only slightly.

3. Switch sides: crunch to the left by lifting your left leg straight up while lowering your right leg as far as is comfortable.

4. Try to do 10 on each side.

Tips

- Try not to pull on your head or neck. Let your abs do the work.

- Try to focus on a slow and controlled movement.

Ways to Challenge Yourself

- Over time, work up to doing 20–30 per side, or to the point of muscle fatigue. (Some people do as many as 50–100 reps per side.) Just be sure to keep good form.

- Instead of resting the lower leg on the floor, try hovering your lowered leg just above the floor without touching it.

- To intensify this exercise, don't put your hands behind your head. Instead, hold light (2- to 5-pound) hand weights. As you crunch to the right, extend your straight left arm to touch your straight right leg as it comes up. Then crunch to the left, touching your straight right arm to your straight left leg.

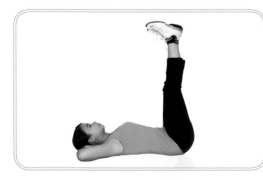 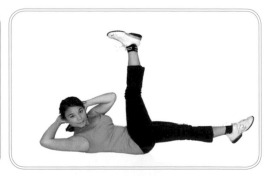

SQUATS

A standard squat is done with both legs in a standing position. To add variety to your routine, we also offer a few variations.

SQUATS WITH MEDICINE BALL

Though I am pictured doing more challenging variation on a balance trainer, feel free to do your squats with no additional equipment. In fact, if you are trying to build strength or power, do your squats from a standing position on the ground, rather than on a balance trainer.

1. Stand with your feet about hip-width apart and your toes pointing forward (*pictured, left*). Engage your core muscles.

2. Keeping your back flat and your head and chest up, squat down by bending your knees as if you're trying to sit down on a chair (*pictured, right*). Visualize your hips/butt moving backward.

3. Return to a standing position while squeezing your butt and thigh muscles.

4. Repeat for about 10 reps.

(*continued*) ▶

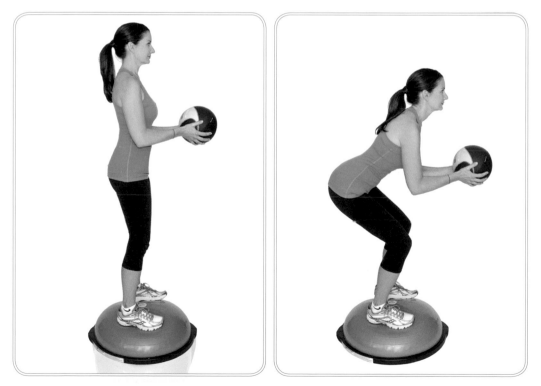

Tips

- If you're new to squats, do them in front of a chair. As you squat down, try to gently touch your bottom to the chair before returning to the standing position. This can help train you to recognize how far to go. But don't worry if you can't quite reach the chair; that's what practice is for!

Ways to Challenge Yourself

- Work up to doing as many as 20–30 squats. Some people do as many as 50–100 squats as part of their workouts; it all depends on your fitness goals and personal health.

- As you increase your strength and stamina, try deepening your squat.

- Standing on a balance trainer (*as pictured*) will help you practice your balance and further engage your muscles as they help you stabilize.

- The resistance from holding a medicine ball as you squat further increases the challenge to your abs.

SUMO SQUAT WITH ROTATION

Feel free to do this squat with no additional equipment. Or, for greater challenge, try holding in both hands a medicine ball or a light to moderate hand weight.

1. Stand with your feet in a wide stance like a sumo wrestler. Your toes should be pointed slightly out with your knees in line with your toes.

2. Keeping your back flat, squat by bending your knees (*pictured, left*). Bring your hands (whether holding equipment or not) toward your waist on your left side.

3. Squeezing your glutes, simultaneously straighten your knees while lifting your hands on a diagonal above your right shoulder (*pictured, right*).

4. Try for 10 reps. Then repeat on the other side.

Ways to Challenge Yourself

- Hold a medicine ball or weight in your hands. In time, work toward holding a heavier weight.

- To really take your squats up a notch, try jump squats—without additional equipment at first. For these do your sumo squat as before, though this time jump upward. Then softly land toes first onto bent knees, sinking back into the sumo squat position. (These are like grand plié ballet jumps, but with less turnout.)

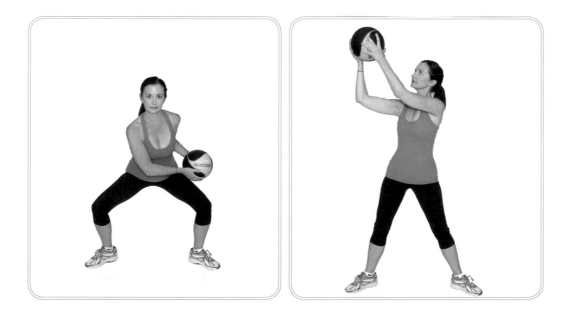

MEDICINE BALL SLAMS

I love medicine ball slams! They're a fun, functional exercise that strengthens the core for movements we make every day. They're also a great way to relieve stress.

Since medicine balls come in different weights, as you build core strength you can graduate to a heavier ball. But feel free to substitute a basketball or similarly sized ball with a good bounce.

1. Stand with feet at least shoulder-width apart or wider.

2. Stiffly engaging your core muscles, lift the ball over your head (*pictured, left*).

3. Keeping your core stiff, simultaneously bend your knees while slamming the ball to the floor (*pictured, right*). The idea is to bounce the ball high enough that you can catch it around hip- or chest-height.

4. Repeat about 10–20 times or until you've had your fun.

Tips

- These are also fun with a partner. Standing about 6–10 feet apart from each other, slam the ball such that it bounces toward your buddy, who'll catch the ball and slam it back to you.

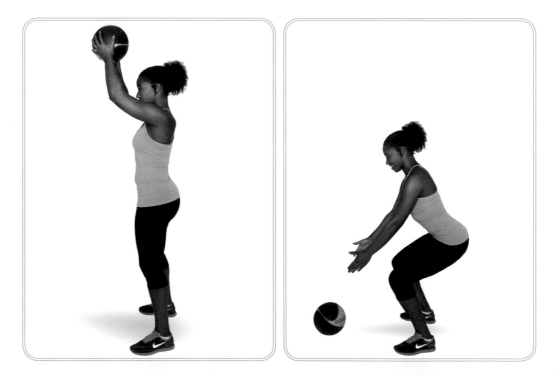

TWIST AND SHOUT!

Twisting exercises, including dancing, are a fun, active, sexy way to engage your core abdominal muscles.

Twists, which involve trunk rotation and engage core abdominal muscles, are common to many exercise programs, including yoga and many popular or classic dances. For one, they're fun! And two, they're very versatile, and can be done on a balance trainer, on an exercise ball, or while standing, sitting, or lying on the floor. Plus, given how often we twist throughout the day—from getting out of bed to switching off the light at night—twist exercises have functional purposes as well. (Note that some exercise scientists recommend we twist from our hips rather than from our spines, so think about leading with your hip.)

RUSSIAN TWISTS

Russian twists, another favorite of mine, engage the oblique muscles. Some women reported experiencing arousal doing this exercise, noting they felt particularly connected to and aware of their core sensations as they twisted back and forth.

1. Sit on the floor with your knees bent at about 90 degrees and your feet flat on the floor. Hold a medicine ball (or some other ball) in front of your chest (*pictured, left*). Keeping your back straight, lean slightly back until you feel your core muscles engage.

2. Squeezing your navel toward your spine, twist to one side, being careful to neither bend nor arch your back (*pictured, right*).

(continued) ▶

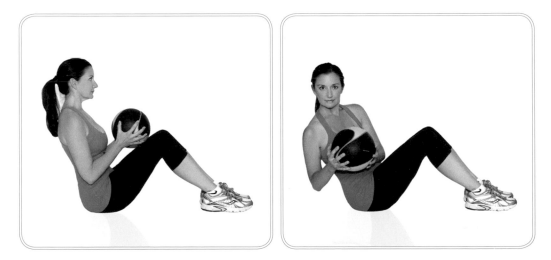

3. In a slow and controlled motion, lead with your hip to twist to the other side, all while breathing in and out.

4. Aim for doing at least 10 on each side. As you get more comfortable, increase your pace as you twist back and forth.

Ways to Challenge Yourself

- Work toward doing 20–30 on each side, or perhaps to the point of muscle fatigue.

- Try raising your feet a few inches off the floor and balancing on your tailbone, as long as you can keep good form.

- Use a small kettleball or a single hand weight in place of a medicine ball.

MEDICINE BALL PASS

Think of this as a Russian twist for two, which makes it even more fun.

1. Start by standing back to back about 6 inches apart from each other. You'll want to keep your knees slightly bent and your core engaged through the entire exercise.

2. One of you should hold a medicine ball at your waist (*pictured, left*).

3. To pass the ball, twist in one direction (say, counterclockwise) as your partner twists in the opposite direction (in this case, clockwise) to receive the ball (*pictured, right*).

4. Once your partner has the ball, she'll then twist counterclockwise to pass the ball to you on the other side, after you've twisted clockwise to meet her.

5. Aim for passing the ball to each other in this manner at least 10 times. Then reverse directions for another 10 passes.

Tips

- You can also do this sitting on the floor, back to back, with your knees bent and feet planted firmly (as with the Russian twist). The passing routine is the same.

- You can also try sitting back to back with your legs outstretched on the floor.

- However you do this, make sure you keep your core engaged throughout.

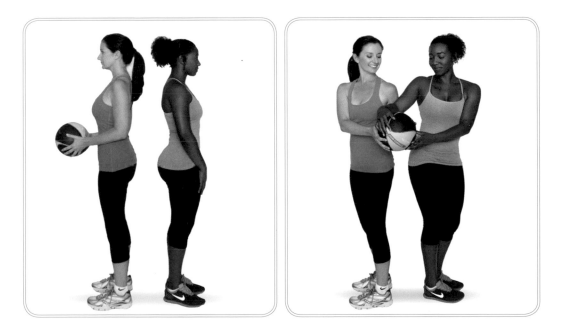

SUPINE BALL TWIST

This rotational exercise doesn't just work the core; it also feels good as it gently massages your back, chest, and arms.

1. Start in a bridge position with your head and shoulders resting on a large stability ball. Your knees should be bent, with your feet planted about hip-width apart on the floor.

2. Make sure to lift your hips so your chest, abs, and thighs form a straight line. Extend your arms above your head with your palms together (*pictured, left*). Stiffen your core.

3. Keeping your feet planted firmly on the floor, slowly and gently roll onto your left shoulder, pointing your outstretched arms to the left (*pictured, right*). (You'll see how keeping your feet in a wide stance keeps you from rolling off the ball.)

4. Next, slowly and gently roll onto your right shoulder, pointing your outstretched arms to the right.

5. Roll back and forth 10 times, breathing in and out.

Ways to Challenge Yourself

- As you become more comfortable and practiced, try for as many as 20–30 reps.

- To challenge your abs, plant your feet closer together. Just be sure not to roll off the ball!

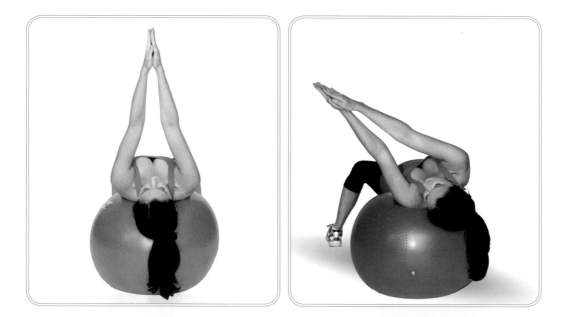

SEATED TWIST

1. Sit on the floor with both legs stretched out in front of you. Plant your right palm on the floor at least 1 foot behind you.

2. Bending your right knee, position your right foot so it's on the left side of your left knee.

3. Now, bending your left arm, position your left elbow to the right side of your bent right knee (*as pictured*). You should feel a stretch in the hip and glute area.

4. Gently push the right knee with your left elbow to increase the stretch. Hold this pose for several breaths.

5. For a nice extra stretch, point and flex the toes of your outstretched leg.

6. Repeat on the opposite side.

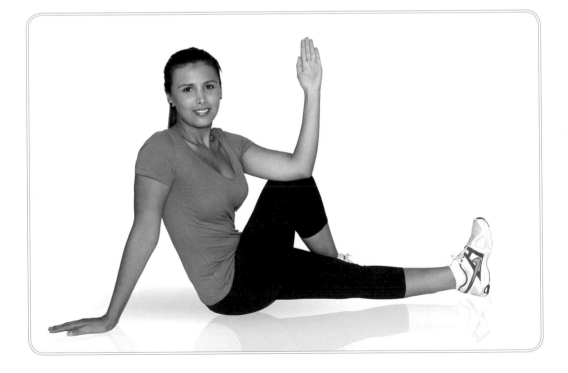

BREATHE . . . AND LIFT UP!

You can also engage your abs with conscious breathing techniques.

Traditional core exercises aren't the only way to work your abs or your greater core. Some research has found core-strengthening benefit in diaphragmatic breathing techniques and pelvic floor activation. In a 2005 study, a certain kind of yoga breathing technique was found to engage core abdominal muscles (particularly the internal and external oblique muscles and the rectus abdominis) even better than traditional crunches do.

Here's the technique:

1. Slowly exhale through the mouth.

2. Next, rapidly inhale through the nose to fully expand the lungs.

3. Now, using the abdominal muscles and the diaphragm as much as possible, quickly exhale through the mouth.

4. After exhaling, keep your mouth closed for about 6 seconds.

As this exercise can be done when seated, it's likely more accessible to those with limited flexibility or other difficulties.

You may recall that some have experienced orgasm from yoga. It's interesting to consider what role their breathing exercises may have played in engaging their core muscles to the point of arousal.

YOUR PELVIC FLOOR

Get to know your pelvic floor muscles.

Remember thinking of the core as a box? Our pelvic floor muscles serve as the bottom of that box. Both Pilates and pelvic floor muscle exercises, which often involve contracting and "lifting" the muscles, have been shown to improve pelvic floor muscle strength in women, which in turn can improve sexual function and orgasmic ability. Further, in a 2008 New Zealand study, researchers found that women who did pelvic floor muscle exercises (such as Kegels) scored significantly better on several measures of sexual experiences than the control group. In other studies, pelvic floor muscle exercises have also been shown to help improve sexual desire and likelihood of orgasm.

Perhaps the most famous pelvic floor muscle exercise is the Kegel. This involves the pubococcygeus muscle (PC muscle), one of several muscles that contract during orgasm and that also controls the flow of urine. (In fact, that's how you can identify the PC muscle: if you can stop the flow of urine, you've found the muscle.) Kegel exercises (detailed below) can help us identify and then strengthen this muscle.

As you get to know your pelvic floor muscles, try to avoid bearing down on them, whether during exercise or when straining with a bowel movement, as it may contribute to muscle weakness and the risk of incontinence. As Dr. Beverly Whipple and Talli Yehuda Rosenbaum write: "Strain during childbirth takes its toll on the PC muscle, and so does age and gravity. Further, many women develop bad habits while exercising that place undue stress on the pelvic floor. It's important to avoid bearing down or pushing these muscles out while lifting weights or practicing aerobics at the gym."

Now, let's set about properly strengthening the PC muscle:

1. Lying on the floor, squeeze the PC muscle for 10 seconds; then relax for 10 seconds. Repeat 10 times. (If at first you can't tighten for 10 seconds, do what you can and then build up slowly.)

2. Next, flutter your PC muscle by contracting and relaxing it as quickly as you can 10 times.

3. Now, try a longer-lasting version. Hold for 10 seconds, then release for 10 seconds.

Note: Ideally, don't "practice" stopping your urine on a regular basis, as doing so can weaken rather than strengthen the muscle.

COREGASM 101

We hope by now you feel you've considered your core and the potential for exercise arousal from every angle. With work and practice, with trial and effort, you'll be able to harness the power of your core to improve your fitness and strength. And with that mastery comes learning to tap into your arousal.

Re-creating Coregasm

We've mentioned that some adults reported having experienced coregasm when they were younger. Many have tried to re-create that arousal, and not always successfully. One of the more inventive strategies for re-creating coregasm came from Anna, who also used to experience orgasms while climbing poles as a child. As a teenager she tried a variety of methods to re-create the feeling, without much luck.

Then one day she stumbled upon a move that worked for her. Sitting on a stool or a chair, with her thighs and knees apart, she places her hands on the chair in between her thighs and pushes against the chair to lift her body off the chair, hovering above it. "It's like I'm flying for sixty seconds," she said.

It's likely the tensing of the lower abdominals and then the lifting of the legs that trigger Anna's arousal. If Anna's invention doesn't work for you, note that a yoga move I call the lotus lift is very similar. (This works best for those who are fairly flexible. For me, lotus is easier when barefoot.)

Stopping Coregasm

Of course, not everyone wants to experience arousal or orgasm during exercise, for a variety of reasons, and that makes sense. Some have expressed not wanting to interrupt their workout, because at times orgasmic feelings can make people feel momentarily tired or weak, as if they couldn't possibly continue. Even many women and men who enjoy feeling exercise arousal don't want to feel these sensations all the time, or in certain contexts. For example, Fawn wrote: "I have a trainer and cannot do push-ups in front of him, as I start to orgasm. He thinks I just can't do them. How can I stop this?"

Given how new this line of research is, there's a lot we don't know. Since we don't yet know definitively what induces arousal, we similarly can't offer surefire methods for avoiding coregasm. But the same suggestions encouraging arousal can be applied, in reverse, to avoid it. As such, listing your non-coregasm options serves as a summary of all that's been conveyed here.

The first step is to **LEARN YOUR OWN PATTERNS**. Become attuned to your bodily sensations so you better understand the variables that bring on arousal. Is it particular exercises or movements? Particularly challenging exercises? A particular order of motions? Once you have a better sense of what drives the arousal, you'll be in a better position to control when and if you encourage it.

For many, the most effective approach was just to **AVOID DOING CERTAIN EXERCISES** in situations where arousal would be uncomfortable. That's what worked for Giana: "The superman exercises cause such a strong physical reaction that I've stopped doing them in public. Having my thighs squeezed tight like that while extending my hips seems to really do it for me!"

Remember the *C* of C.O.R.E.? "Challenge yourself." So the next arousal-stoppers concern various ways to make the **EXERCISE LESS CHALLENGING**. This might include **SLOWING YOUR PACE** if your arousal begins when you're running, biking, or swimming, or **REDUCING THE INTENSITY** of your movements. If you're doing ab exercises, do fewer; or do them in sets, with rests in between. If you're doing strength training, choose a less challenging weight. Just as there are many means of increasing the intensity of your workout, you have a range of options for reducing it too.

> I generally get a "runners high" and then get fairly aroused when I've run more than a couple miles. After a few miles I can often orgasm by contracting my pelvic floor muscles several times in quick succession. Occasionally I'll orgasm just from running without trying; if I feel that coming on I can usually stop it by slowing down or changing my gait.
>
> I generally just stop what I'm doing, as the strength of my orgasm would make it impossible to hide what is happening.

Of course, another means of decreasing the likelihood of arousal takes the opposite approach: **BUILD YOUR ENDURANCE** so it's harder to challenge yourself. As you may recall, some people found that as they got stronger, their coregasms took more work to bring on. Fawn, who couldn't do push-ups in front of her trainer without orgasming, found a solution: she practiced push-ups at home to build up her endurance. In time, she was able to do them at the gym with her trainer without reaching orgasm. Of course, building strength often makes it *easier* to experience coregasm overall. Since this works differently for different people, you'll want to monitor your own experience.

Another approach is to experiment with **DIFFERENT BREATHING PATTERNS** to see if a change in breathing influences feelings of arousal. Some women learned that if they held their breath or started breathing very slowly, they were able to delay or completely stop their coregasm.

Recall that mindfulness is key to many women's experiences of arousal or orgasm. Just as distraction can inhibit sexual arousal, **DISTRACTING YOURSELF** can be an effective buzz-kill in the gym as well. One woman who experiences orgasms during many different exercises noticed that she never experienced orgasm during group exercise classes. She reasoned that paying close attention to the instructors, as well as continually comparing her form with that of others in the class, suppressed her arousal.

For some, the guidance to *relax and receive* ends up being the best approach. Many have found it's just easier to be receptive to the feelings, to pause and **LET THEM PASS**. Then, after a few moments, they can continue working out.

I've been exercising for most of my life. You name it, I've done it: yoga, weights, Pilates, running, swimming, dance classes, team sports. I never noticed any arousal before until I made the changes you suggested. I think what did it was a combination of the exercises themselves and me learning to pay attention to my body and not push those feelings away. Doing the ab exercises to fatigue definitely paid off! I also liked learning more core exercises than I knew before. I feel more powerful as a woman knowing how to create arousal in my own body whenever I want.

—GABRIELA

COREGASM 101 ADVANCED AB CHALLENGE

Some women in our research—particularly very strong or fit women—found it took quite a bit to challenge their abs. And some found it wasn't adding reps that did the trick, but adding difficulty. If this is the case for you, note that these more demanding exercises have proven effective for many coregasmic women:

- Bicycle crunches

- Chin-ups

- Pull-ups

- Hanging leg raises

Remember Rose, who skips cardio to save her energy for pull-ups? Rose does nine pull-ups in a row to induce her coregasm. (And note: nine pull-ups is a lot! I've never managed even one unassisted pull-up.) She knows her body well enough to have perfected this technique. After the ninth pull-up, she switches to a bar hang, then lifts her knees up to her chest: this produces the best feeling for her.

It so happens that Rose discovered on her own what some researchers concluded in a study: "The most demanding exercise is pelvic tilting with the knees and hips bent while hanging from a chin-up bar." So be your own research student: discover what works best for you.

7

It was never intentional. Arousal would usually happen about forty minutes into a kickboxing aerobics class.

—HAILEY

CHAPTER 7

THE COREGASM WORKOUT EXERCISES AND ROUTINES

WE ALL KNOW that exercising regularly—and often—is important to our overall health. Both the American Health Association and the American College of Sports Medicine recommend that adults engage in strength exercises using all our major muscle groups at least twice a week. Twice a week can be considered "regularly." But exercising often—more than twice a week—also helps many people reach their fitness goals. Most women and men who are training for a running race, from a 5K to a marathon, train by running several days a week, steadily increasing their mileage leading up to the race length by race time. Building muscle generally calls for strength training at least two or three days a week. Remember that with weight training rest days (with no exercise) or days with easier workouts are essential for giving your muscles time to recover.

Regular workouts have other benefits too. A 2013 study found that college students who work out more often have been shown to have higher grades. Exercising regularly— at least three times a week at a moderate intensity—has been shown to improve mood and lower symptoms of depression. And a 2014 study found that women who work out between two and three-plus times per week have higher bone density than women who work out less often.

Despite all these benefits, which are not well-kept secrets, unfortunately most of us don't get enough exercise. The U.S. government recommends that women and men get at least 150 minutes of moderate-to-intense aerobic exercise, or at least 75 minutes of vigorous-to-intense exercise, or some combination of these *each week*. Plus, it's recommended we incorporate muscle-strengthening activities like core-strengthening or weight lifting exercises into our routines at least twice a week. Think about the past week—did you get enough exercise?

If your answer is no, you are not alone. A 2013 report from the U.S. Centers for Disease Control and Prevention found that *only about 20 percent* of Americans met these fitness goals! Are you ready to join me in exercising more often and meeting our fitness goals? Both aerobic and strength exercise?

By now you've likely encountered quite a few of the thirty-plus exercises in this book. Perhaps you've even tried some of them. But even if you haven't, please don't let the number "thirty-plus" discourage you, as no one expects you to do thirty exercises in one workout—I certainly don't. The exercises in the Coregasm Workout were all selected to help you build a stronger core and to enhance your overall health and fitness—and with so many to choose from, you're likely to find some that work for you, with enough variety to keep your workouts fresh and fun. As the saying goes, if you have fun when you work out, it won't feel like work. And the Coregasm Workout can definitely be fun.

This program combines certain exercises and certain ways of exercising to help you become more in touch with your body and its sensations—in a manner that's also safe and healthy. If you want to experience greater arousal while exercising, and connect with your body and its sensations in this way, then I invite you to try. It may take several weeks or months. Like any workout, it will take time, dedication, and a commitment to core exercise. However, I believe in you and I believe in this program.

Of course, everyone has different health needs, and we're all built a little differently. That's why I designed the Coregasm Workout to be easily tailored to individual goals and concerns. I encourage you to consult medical professionals and fitness experts to help you craft what works best for you. Particularly if you have back pain or health concerns, or if you're pregnant or recovering from an injury, you should ask a doctor, nurse, or physical therapist before beginning any new exercise program, including this one.

Also, if you have questions about exercising (including how to adjust exercises in safe ways for you), a physical therapist or a personal trainer can be an excellent person to talk with. In the U.S., some of the more recognized certifying bodies are the American College of Sports Medicine (ACSM), the American Council on Exercise (ACE), the National Strength and Conditioning Association (NSCA), and the Aerobic and Fitness Association of America (AFAA).

As you tailor the Coregasm Workout for your own body and fitness goals, try to keep the C.O.R.E. Principles in mind.

C: Challenge yourself.
O: Order matters.
R: Relax and receive.
E: Engage your lower abs.

Also, consider doing both aerobic exercise ("cardio") and strength-training exercise. And, of course, to help improve or maintain flexibility, remember to warm up before you begin and stretch after you're done. Life is long, and you deserve a healthy, fit, strong, and flexible body to help you do all the things you want to do with it for as long as you can.

CARDIO EXERCISE

Aerobic exercise is cardiovascular exercise, which benefits the heart. If you're planning on light-to-moderate exercise, the idea is to get your heart rate up but still be able to carry on a conversation. This is definitely the pace to aim for if you're just starting. Once you're ready for a more intense or challenging workout, say with sprints, for example, increase your exertion such that carrying on a conversation would be difficult, if not impossible.

If you choose to include aerobic exercise in your workout, as discussed earlier, you have a range of options to choose from. The important thing is to get moving—so find what feels right to you and try to keep at it for at least 20 to 30 minutes if possible. (If you need to go slow; that's fine. Do what you can—10 minutes is a good initial goal—and try to build up over time.) And for those more advanced exercisers, try for as long as 45 to 60 minutes or more.

Cardio Exercises

Not sure what might count as cardio? Here are some ideas to get started:

GENERAL

- Biking
- Dancing
- Golfing
- Hiking
- Rock climbing
- Roller skating
- Running
- Walking
- Water aerobics
- Yoga

Plus, playing:

- Basketball
- Frisbee
- Hockey
- Kickball
- Soccer
- Softball/baseball
- Tennis
- Volleyball

AT THE GYM

- Aerobic dance class
- Aerobic step class
- Elliptical trainer or cross-trainer
- High-intensity interval training (H.I.I.T.)
- Kettleball
- Kickboxing
- Stairclimber
- Stationary biking/"spin class" cycle workout
- Treadmill (walking or running)

AT HOME

- Jogging in place
- Jumping jacks
- Marching in place
- Mopping
- Mowing the lawn with a push mower
- Playing tag with your kids
- Raking
- Sweeping
- Walking the dog
- Walking the kids to and from school or bus stop

WATER ACTIVITIES

- Canoeing
- Kayaking
- Paddleboarding
- Surfing
- Swimming
- Water aerobics
- Water skiing
- Windsurfing

WINTER ACTIVITIES

- Cross-country skiing
- Downhill skiing
- Ice skating
- Shoveling snow
- Snowshoeing

Challenge Your Cardio

Remember: C.O.R.E. Principle 1 is to challenge yourself. So keep that in mind for whatever aerobic exercise you choose. Here's how you might challenge yourself through cardio:

- If you're going on a walk, try walking briskly; or mix up your walk by including a 30-second jogging burst every few minutes. Or occasionally try jogging with your dog.

- If you're swimming, every few laps pretend you're in the Olympics and give it your best effort.

- On a treadmill, try increasing the incline on your walk or jog or use the preprogrammed interval option.

- If you normally use a cardio machine at the gym, try exercising at one level higher than usual.

- Toss a Frisbee with a friend, but don't go easy; challenge yourselves by tossing a little farther or to the side so you have to run.

- Join a kickball team! Run hard from base to base!

COREGASM WORKOUT EXERCISES

Remember: this workout program focuses first on helping your overall core strength and fitness—and if you discover arousal along the way, then that's great too. But the "core" comes first, then the "gasm." And while many have reported experiencing exercise arousal or orgasm from certain exercises in this program, that's not the case for all the exercises and stretches included here. Rather, the exercises were chosen because—overall—they provide a range of ways for you to strengthen your core, work toward better balance, and generally aim for feeling fit and healthy.

Keep the C.O.R.E. Principles in mind as you go through each exercise. Try to **CHALLENGE YOURSELF** to get the best workout possible. When it comes to reps, you may want to start out at beginner levels. As you become stronger and more fit, try to increase your reps. You may even want to work out continuously (doing all at once your reps of a particular exercise) rather than in sets. Whatever you do, just make sure to keep good form; if you notice your form slipping, it may be time to stop and rest a little bit before continuing. Over time, you'll feel stronger and ready to go deeper into your workouts.

If you want to enhance your arousal while working out, then remember that **ORDER MATTERS**; this means you may want to do cardio before working your abs. Also, if you notice some arousal emerging during a certain exercise, consider building on that arousal with another intense ab exercise. Try to relax and focus your mind. If you happen to notice feelings of arousal, consider **RELAXING INTO RECEIVING** those feelings.

Finally, some of these exercises target and **ENGAGE THE LOWER ABDOMINAL MUSCLES**, so try to balance your routine with lower ab work.

Again, this program was designed to help you feel stronger, fitter, and healthier—all of which can contribute to feeling sexier as well. I hope you enjoy the Coregasm Workout!

INDIVIDUAL CORE EXERCISES

Remember: In between exercises, you may want to get or keep your heart rate up. This could involve marching or jogging in place, doing jumping jacks, jumping up and down, hopping on one foot—even skipping across the room for extra fun. These kinds of cardio and quick intervals help some women to connect more easily with arousal. I often do ten jumping jacks or jog in place between strength-training exercises.

Warm-Up

Regardless of your fitness level, the cat/cow and bridge poses will gently let your core know it's time to work!

CAT/COW

The cat/cow posture is common to many yoga classes, and is sometimes used in childhood dance classes. It's a great warm-up since it gently moves the spine.

1. Begin on all fours in a "tabletop" position. Your hands should be directly beneath your shoulders, your knees directly beneath your hips. Your spine should be in a neutral position—in a relatively straight line from your head to your hips. It may help to think of having a long neck (*pictured, top*). Your gaze should be toward the floor.

2. On an inhale, move into cow pose by lifting your sitting bones up, gently lifting your chest and chin, and gazing toward the ceiling. Some people choose to curl their toes under as well. Try to move slowly and gently, with your neck the last part to move (*pictured, bottom left*).

3. On an exhale, move into cat by rounding your spine, tucking your tailbone, and dropping your head; your gaze should be toward the floor or your navel (*pictured, bottom right*).

4. Alternate between cow pose and cat pose about 10 times in slow, fluid movements. Be sure to consistently inhale for cow pose and exhale for cat pose.

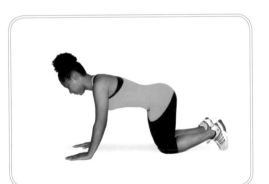

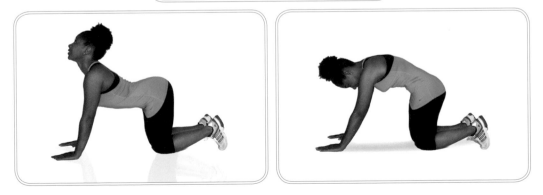

BRIDGE

Bridge is another pose that's gentle on the spine, which makes it ideal both toward the beginning and toward the end of a workout session.

1. Lie on your back with your knees bent and your arms on the floor alongside your body (*pictured, left*). Your feet should be flat on the floor with your heels close to your sitting bones. Palms can be flat or facing up.

2. On an exhale, press your feet and arms into the floor as you squeeze your buttocks and core abdominal muscles, thus lifting your hips off the floor (*pictured, right*). Your thighs should be parallel and your knees should be over your heels.

3. Try to maintain core engagement (continue squeezing) for as long as you hold this pose.

4. If you are comfortable in the pose and would like to take it deeper, clasp your hands together on the mat underneath your body.

5. Stay in the pose for at least 5 breath cycles. As you become more comfortable in the pose, try to build up to holding the bridge for about 10 breath cycles.

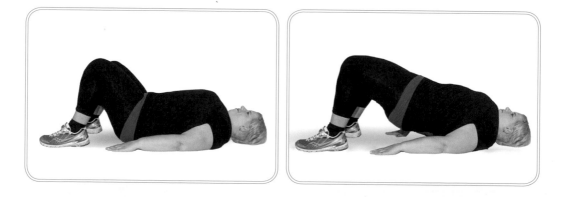

To aim for a balanced exercise program, here is some guidance on how many exercises to choose from each section and which exercises may be better for beginners, intermediate exercises, or those who are more advanced—keeping in mind that you and your healthcare provider know your body best.

Core Abdominal Exercises

Beginners might want to start with prone plank and crunches. Intermediate exercisers might choose two from prone plank, crunches, or leg raises. More advanced exercisers can choose three exercises from prone plank, crunches, leg raises, stability ball knee tuck, or stability ball pass.

Core Abdominal Exercises with Rotation

If you're a beginner, start with either bicycle crunches or Russian twists (just choose one at first). More intermediate exercisers can choose two exercises from bicycle crunches, Russian twists, side planks, or extended bicycle crunches. And if you're advanced? Choose two from bicycle crunches, Russian twists, side planks, extended bicycle crunches, or supine ball twist.

Core

Beginners, start with supine plank and/or superman. Intermediate and advanced levels might also want to try the swimmer.

PRONE PLANK

Modeled on the push-up, plank exercises have become very popular in recent years, and are often considered an essential part of core fitness programs. Though planks may look simple, they require constant, active engagement of a number of core muscles, which can help build a strong core.

1. Start by lying facedown on the floor with your palms touching the floor directly beneath your shoulders. Your core should be tight.

2. Push/lift yourself into a bent-knee push-up or a standard push-up.

   BENT-KNEE VARIATION: Your knees remain touching the floor, your calves and feet in the air behind you. This variation can make planks easier to incorporate into your workout since it requires your core to support less of your body weight. Your body should be in a straight line from your head to your knees.

   STANDARD (STRAIGHT) LEG: Keep your legs straight with the balls of your feet on the floor. They can be planted wide apart (which is easier) or closer together (which is more challenging).

3. Your body should form a relatively straight line, either from your head to your knees (bent-knee variation) or from your head to your feet (straight-leg variation). Holding your abs in will make it easier to stay in plank, so try to keep your back flat, pulling your belly button toward your spine (as pictured).

4. For more muscle engagement, squeeze your glutes and engage your quads as if you're drawing your kneecaps up toward your thighs.

5. Breathe in and out.

6. If you're new to plank, try to stay in the plank position for about 10 seconds. As you build strength and comfort, work up to holding for 30 seconds, then for 1 minute. Some people work toward holding planks for several minutes. Do what feels right for you!

Ways to Challenge Yourself

- Advance from bent-knee to standard plank.

- Bring your feet closer together.

- Hold the position longer—even up to 4 minutes, if you can!

- Lift one leg (or one arm) off the ground.

- Instead of having your hands on the floor, plank with your forearms and elbows on the floor. Your forearms should completely touch the floor, with your elbows directly beneath your shoulders.

- Plank on a large exercise ball instead of on the ground, resting your forearms on the ball. You should feel your body working to balance and stabilize itself.

(For the supine plank, see page 103.)

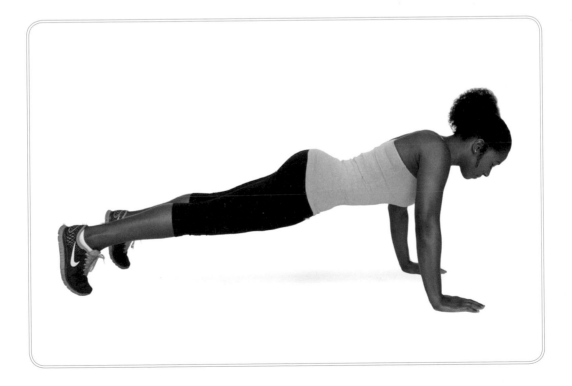

BICYCLE CRUNCHES

Bicycle crunches are a common core exercise that effectively engages several abdominal muscles. They can be arousal-inducing as well; bicycle crunches are some women's primary coregasmic exercise.

1. Lie on your back with your knees bent and feet planted on the floor, about hip-width apart.

2. Start by drawing your right knee toward your chest and straightening your left leg as you crunch forward, drawing your left elbow toward your right knee (*as pictured*). Your left elbow and shoulder blade should come just a few inches off the floor.

3. Now reverse the move: straighten your right leg and draw your left knee toward your chest as you crunch forward, drawing your right elbow toward your left knee. This time your right elbow and shoulder blade will come just a few inches off the floor.

4. Keep alternating sides. Aim for at least 10 crunches in each direction; eventually, try to work up to 20 to 30 on each side, or to the point of muscle fatigue.

Tips

- Do not pull on your neck and do not push your head with your hands. Your abs should be doing the work here.

- Try to focus on a slow and controlled movement.

Ways to Challenge Yourself

- If you've developed a strong core and can keep going with good form, try continuing bicycle crunches to the point of fatigue. For some women this can be as many as 50 to 100 (or more) crunches per side.

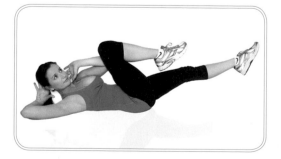

LEG RAISES

Leg raises—whether done lying on the floor, as pictured here, or on a Captain's Chair/Roman Chair at the gym—commonly lead to arousal for some women. Leg raises on the floor are easier and safer than those done on a Captain's Chair/Roman Chair, which are best attempted with a trainer to ensure proper form.

1. Lying on your back, lift your legs in the air until they are perpendicular to your body, about a 90-degree angle (*pictured, left*).

2. While keeping your abs tight and your navel pulled in toward your spine, very slowly lower your legs toward the floor in a smooth and controlled motion (*pictured, right*). Press your back into the floor while lowering your legs down toward the floor, but stop before your feet reach the floor.

3. Lift your legs back to the starting position and repeat. Aim to do 10 reps at first; over time, work to complete 20–30 reps.

Tips

- Make sure your lower back stays on the floor. If you feel your lower back arching or coming off the floor, don't lower your legs any farther. That may be a good stopping place for you.

- As you continue to do core exercises more regularly, you may develop enough strength to eventually lower your legs closer to the floor.

Ways to Challenge Yourself

- As you grow stronger and build endurance, it may take more reps to get you to the point of fatigue—perhaps as many as 50–100 leg raises.

- To mix it up and keep it interesting, do single leg raises instead of lifting and lowering both at once.

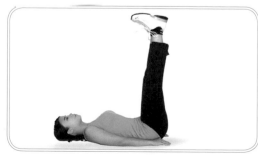 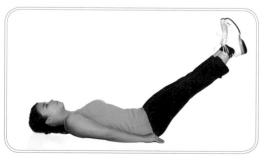

SUPERMAN

Superman is good for your core, glutes, hamstrings, and lower back. Many people neglect lower back exercises, but they are an important part of core training. Plus, given its motion of squeezing and tensing the body, Superman is also an exercise that some find particularly arousing.

1. Start by lying on your stomach with your arms extended in front of you and your legs stretched behind you, feet apart (*pictured, top*).

2. Keeping your arms and legs straight and your core fully engaged and tight, all at once raise your arms, chest, and feet a few inches off the floor by stretching your arms out and squeezing your butt and thighs together (*pictured, bottom*). Continue to breathe in and out.

3. Try to hold this pose for 10 seconds at first, then release and relax. Try to repeat 2–3 times.

Tips

- At first you may be able to lift your upper and lower body only an inch or two off the ground. That's okay. With practice you can increase your core strength, and over time may be able to lift higher.

Ways to Challenge Yourself

- Over time, work toward holding this pose for 30–60 seconds, then release.

- Or, rather than holding it for a length of time, increase your reps, up to 20–30, but holding for just 1 or 2 seconds each.

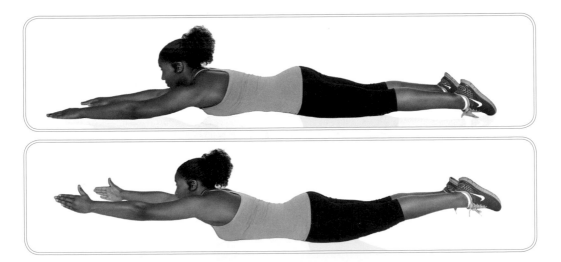

SWIMMER

The swimmer is another core exercise that is particularly beneficial for the backside of the body: glutes, hamstrings, and lower back.

1. Start by lying on your stomach with your arms stretched above your head and your legs straight.

2. Keeping your limbs straight, simultaneously lift your chest and left arm and your right leg at least several inches off the floor (*as pictured*). Aim for keeping your movements fluid and your breathing steady.

3. Switch to working the opposite limbs: lift your chest and right arm and your left leg at least several inches off the floor.

4. Continue alternating sides, breathing and fluidly moving your limbs as if you were swimming.

5. Try to do at least 10 on each side, building up to 20–30 per side or until fatigued.

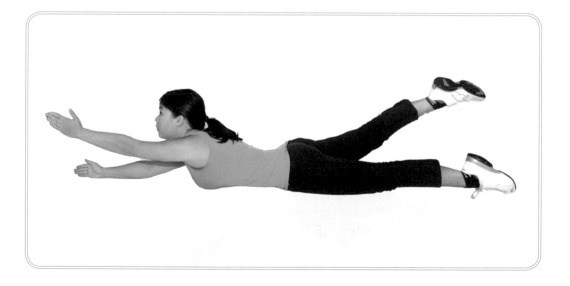

STABILITY BALL KNEE TUCK

This (very) advanced move is also a fun one!

1. Begin in the starting position for downward-facing dog but with a large exercise ball beneath you. Slowly walk your hands out away from the ball until your shins are resting on the ball and your body is extended (*pictured, left*).

2. You should be basically in a plank position—with your body straight and parallel to the floor—just with your shins on the ball. Your hands should be planted on the floor, palms down, your wrists and hands directly beneath your shoulders. Look straight down at the floor.

3. Squeezing your abs and keeping your legs active, use your feet to roll the ball toward you, pulling your knees toward your chest, stopping just under your hips (*pictured, right*). Try to keep your shoulders straight. Your knees should be under your hips. Hold this position for one breath, then return to the plank position by rolling the ball back.

4. Repeat if you can. At first you may be able to do this only one or two times. With practice and patience—and possibly a few accidental slips off the ball—you should be able in time to build up to 10 or even 20 reps.

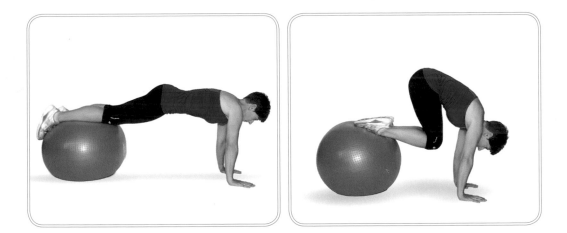

STABILITY BALL PASS

This is another fun core exercise, though it takes a little coordination. Be patient with yourself.

1. With a large exercise ball in your hands, begin by lying on the floor with your arms stretched above your head and your feet shoulder-width apart (*pictured, top*).

2. Keeping your limbs outstretched, lift your arms and legs to meet, with the ball in your hands now above your body. "Hugging" the ball on either side with your feet, transfer/ pass the ball from your hands to your feet (*pictured, middle*).

3. With the ball now secured by your feet, lower your arms and legs back toward the floor (*pictured, bottom*).

4. Repeat the process in reverse, returning the ball to your hands.

5. Try for at least 10 reps of passing the ball to your feet and returning it to your hands.

Tips

- Work to press your lower back toward the floor with this exercise. If you feel your lower back arching, don't lower your arms and legs quite so far.

Ways to Challenge Yourself

- Repeat at least 20 times or until fatigued. Some people love this exercise and do as many as 40 or more reps. Maybe you will too!

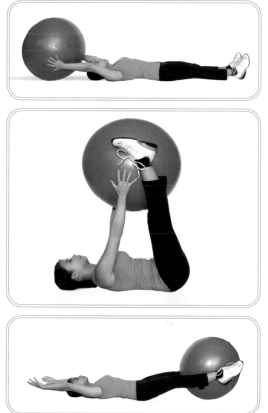

STRENGTH TRAINING

No program is complete without a little strength training! It's important to build and maintain strength so we stay healthy and fit doing all the different motions we do in life, from emptying the washing machine to moving an entire household.

If your goal is to build more power and strength, then you might not want to use a balance trainer when lifting weights. Instead, stick with the stable floor or bench. But if balance is more your goal, then working on a balance trainer for certain exercises might be a good choice for you. Regardless, be sure to discuss your options with a fitness or health expert, as there are different approaches to resistance/weight training.

UPPER BODY: If you're a beginner, choose two exercises from the following: push-ups, medicine ball slams, medicine ball passes, medicine ball circles, biceps curls, and triceps extensions. If you're an intermediate exerciser, choose three exercises from the same list. Advanced? Choose four.

LOWER BODY: If you're a beginner, choose two, multidirectional lunges, skater jumps, or tree pose. If you're intermediate, squats with a medicine ball are an option (choose three exercises). If you're advanced, choose four of these exercises.

PUSH-UPS

"Drop and give me 10!" Many of us first tried doing some form of push-up when we were kids. A push-up is a classic core exercise that also engages various muscles in the chest and back. For some, they can also induce arousal.

To follow, we offer steps for the two most common push-ups: the push-up from the knee and the standard push-up. Freddie (*pictured*) is demonstrating the standard push-up on an overturned balance trainer.

1. Start by lying facedown on the floor with your palms touching the floor directly beneath your shoulders. Your core should be tight.

   BENT-KNEE VARIATION: Bend your knees so your calves and feet are in the air behind you. Your knees remain touching the floor.

2. With your feet (or knees) still touching the floor, and keeping your eyes focused on the floor, in a slow and controlled motion straighten your arms to push/lift yourself into a push-up (*pictured, left*). Note that your body should be in a straight line from your head to your feet (or from your head to your knees if you're doing the bent-knee variation).

3. In a slow and controlled motion, bend your elbows so that you lower your chest and chin close to the floor without fully reaching it (*pictured, right*). Make sure to keep your abs tight (drawing your navel toward your spine) throughout the push-up. Keep your body in a straight line.

4. Repeat the process, aiming for a few push-ups, if possible.

(*continued*) ▶

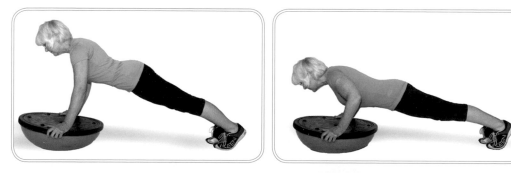

Tips

- At first you may be able to do just a few push-ups—or even just one. That's okay! Push-ups are a difficult exercise that uses your body weight for resistance.
- Over time you can build up to 10, then 20, then 30 or more.

Ways to Challenge Yourself

- Graduate from knee push-ups to standard push-ups.
- Once you're comfortable with standard push-ups, adjust how wide apart you plant your feet: wide apart is easier; closer together is more challenging.
- For a change of pace or to work on your balance, try push-ups on a balance trainer, as Freddie (*pictured*) is doing.

MEDICINE BALL CIRCLES

Though Bianca (*pictured*) is challenging herself by standing on a balance trainer, feel free to do these just standing on the floor.

1. Holding a medicine ball, stand with your arms extended in front of you (*pictured, left*).

2. Circle your arms clockwise around you in a slow and controlled motion (*pictured, right*). Return to facing forward. Repeat this 10 times.

3. Switch directions, now circling your arms 10 times counterclockwise.

Ways to Challenge Yourself

- Build up to doing 20–30 circles in each direction.

- Increase the weight of the medicine ball you're using.

- Standing on a balance trainer helps you practice your balance and may engage your core abdominal muscles in different ways than on the ground.

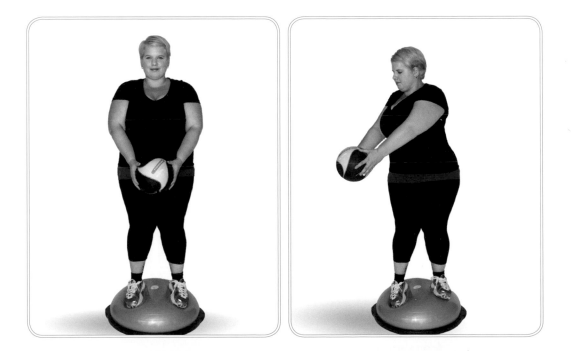

SKATER JUMPS

Skater jumps engage the core and work the lower body while also upping heart rate. (You can do these with or without holding a medicine ball.)

1. Start in a wide stance with your knees slightly bent. Keeping your back straight, hinge slightly forward from your hips. If you choose to use a medicine ball, hold it comfortably in front of you (*pictured, left*).

2. Leading with your right foot, jump laterally (to the side); your left foot should follow your right foot, coming down behind your right heel in a curtsy-type pose (*pictured, right*). Note: when you jump to the side, try to land with a soft, bent knee.

3. Repeat on the other side, each time landing in the curtsy position with a soft, bent knee.

4. Aim for 10 jumps on each side.

Tips

- Go slowly until you get the hang of the rhythm and moves. With just a little practice, the exercise will come more naturally and more quickly.

Ways to Challenge Yourself

- Work up to 20 jumps on each side.

- If you work with a medicine ball, hold it throughout the exercise, allowing it to lead you at the end of each leap into a slight twist toward the outside hip. This extra twist will help further engage your side abdominal muscles.

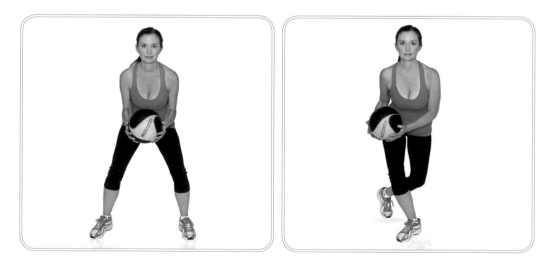

BICEPS CURLS

1. Stand on the floor or on a balance trainer with your feet about hip-width apart and your knees slightly bent. Holding a weight in each hand, let your arms hang down at your sides, your palms facing forward (*pictured, top*).

2. Tighten your abs, pulling your navel toward your spine.

3. Bending your elbows and keeping them close to your body, curl the weights upward until your hands reach your shoulders (*pictured, bottom*). This works the full range of motion for your biceps.

4. Lower the weights to your starting position. Try to use slow and controlled movements, breathing slowly in and out.

5. Repeat, aiming for 10 reps with each arm.

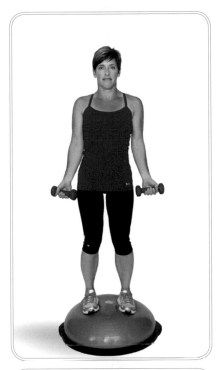

Tips

- Remember to use slow and controlled movements, breathing slowly in and out.

- Start with a light, comfortable weight. Though you can slowly increase your weights as you build strength, don't try to advance too quickly.

Ways to Challenge Yourself

- As you build strength, aim for 30 or more reps per side, or to the point of fatigue.

- You can do these reps continuously (30 in a row) or discontinuously (three sets of 10 reps each).

- Do fewer reps using a heavier weight.

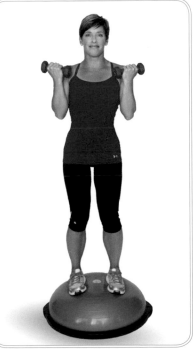

TRICEPS EXTENSIONS

Your triceps are an important but often overlooked muscle in the arm that can sag as we age. Tricep extensions can help to keep these muscles toned.

1. Stand on the floor or on an balance trainer holding a weight in each hand and with knees slightly bent.

2. Keeping your hands parallel and palms facing one another, raise your arms straight above your head (*pictured, top*).

3. Keeping your elbows pointing forward, slowly lower the weights behind your head by bending your elbows (*pictured, bottom*). Work to keep your movements slow and controlled and your breathing steady.

4. Being careful to not knock your head with the weights, return to starting position.

5. Try to do a total of 10 reps. Over time, you may be able to build up to 20–30 reps.

Tips

- Remember to keep your movements slow and controlled, mindfully breathing in and out.

- You can also do this exercise from a seated position. Just be sure to keep your back straight and your abs squeezed in tight.

- Some people find it easier to exercise one arm at a time. Don't feel like that's the easy way out, though; some research suggests exercising one arm at a time can build more strength.

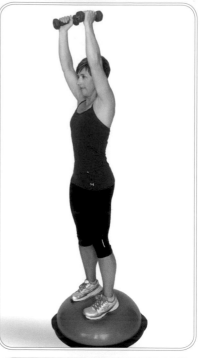

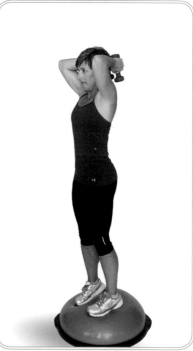

MULTIDIRECTIONAL LUNGES

Forward Lunges

1. Stand with your feet about hip-width apart (*pictured, top*). Keep your back straight.

2. Lunge forward by planting your right foot firmly in front of you, with your knee at a 90-degree angle directly above your ankle. Make sure your knee doesn't extend over your toes—you should be able to see your toes. (Note that the *bottom* picture shows Freddie in a deep lunge, which is advanced. Don't worry if you can't yet sink as deeply; you'll get there with time and practice.)

3. Reverse the process to return to the starting position. Repeat on the other side, alternating legs to complete 10–20 forward lunges on each side.

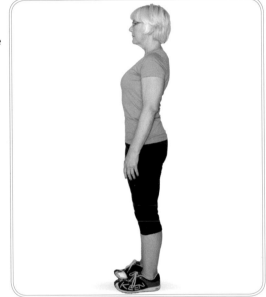

Reverse Lunges

1. To do reverse lunges, start from the same place, standing tall with your feet about hip-width apart.

2. Simply step backward instead of forward. Plant the ball of your foot on the floor behind you and sink into a lunge, keeping your back straight. Look at your front foot to make sure that your knee and ankle are in a straight line, with your knee at a 90-degree angle.

3. Push forward and return to the starting position. Repeat on the other side, alternating legs to complete 10–20 backward lunges on each side.

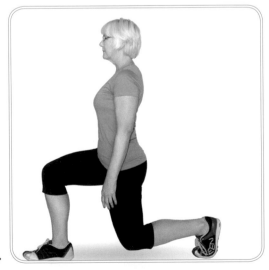

(continued) ▶

Side Lunges

1. Begin by standing on the floor with your feet about hip-width apart, both pointing forward.

2. This time step out to the side, planting your foot as you bend into your lunge: one leg bent, one leg straight. Holding your head high above your shoulders, keep your torso straight, your head and chest up, and your posture tall.

3. Return to the starting position and repeat on the other side. Alternate legs to complete 10–20 lunges on each side.

Around-the-World Lunges

With around-the-world lunges you do one in each direction in one big circle.

1. Stand with your feet hip-width apart.

2. Lunge forward with your right foot and return to starting position.

3. Lunge to the side with your right foot and return to starting position.

4. Do a reverse lunge with your right foot; return to starting position.

5. Now it's time to switch. This time, do a reverse lunge with your left foot; return to starting position.

6. Lunge to the left side with your left foot; return to starting position.

7. Do your last lunge forward with your left foot; return to starting position.

8. This was one complete rotation "around the world." Aim for 5 total rotations.

Ways to Challenge Yourself

- If you find these aren't challenging enough, intensify the exercise by holding hand weights. Just be sure you don't sacrifice your form: back straight, knee and ankle in alignment, gaze straight ahead.

COOL-DOWN STRETCHES

Beginners can choose three from downward-facing dog, three-legged dog, quad stretch, butterfly, or seated twist. Intermediate and advanced exercisers can choose three from downward-facing dog, three-legged dog, butterfly, seated twist, or pigeon.

BUTTERFLY

After you've had a good workout, it's important to stretch your inner thigh muscles. The butterfly—which I remember doing in preschool ballet classes—is a great way to stretch your muscles in a seated position.

1. This stretch is very simple. Just sit on the floor with your knees bent to the sides and the soles of your feet together.

2. Note that most people's knees like mine, (*pictured*) will not touch the floor in this position; please don't give knee-touching a moment's thought. Your knees may be even higher off the ground; that's common! This is also not a glamorous pose, and it tends to make our bellies and thighs appear more squishy than they really are. So please practice loving kindness toward your body. It takes care of you every day!

3. Breathe in and out, keeping your back straight and your gaze forward. If you like, bend forward at the hips/waist to increase the stretch. Try to hold this pose for 10 slow and gentle breaths.

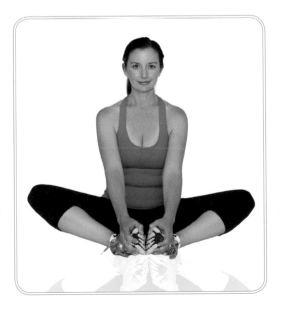

QUAD STRETCH

1. Stand with your feet planted on the floor, about hip-width apart. Look straight ahead of you.

2. Bend your right knee to lift your right foot behind you, taking it in your hand.

3. Try to keep your knees close to each other and your legs parallel. To increase the stretch, think of pushing your shoelaces into your hand.

4. Hold this stretch for several breaths—to a count of 20 if possible—and return to starting position.

5. Repeat on the other side.

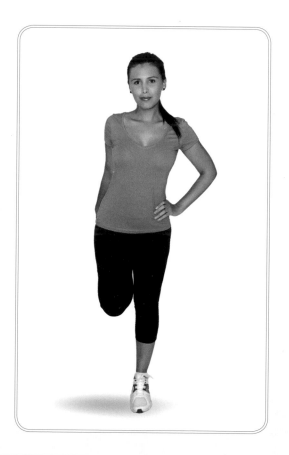

SAMPLE WORKOUTS

To follow you'll find different Coregasm Workout routines in a range of fitness levels, plus an all-level workout for the gym. With this variety you can tailor any day's workout to your energy level, inspiration, and environment—whether you're exercising at home, outdoors, or at the gym.

Sample Beginner Workout

CARDIO

Warm up for 5–10 minutes by walking, marching, or jogging in place.

EXERCISES

Cat/cow (page 129)

Bridge (page 130)

Prone plank (page 132)

Crunches (page 104)

Russian twists (page 111)

Superman (page 136)

Swimmer (page 137)

Push-ups from knees on floor (page 141)

Medicine ball circles, from a standing position on floor (page 143)

Squats, with or without a medicine ball (page 107)

Lunges (page 147)

Downward-facing dog (page 85)

Quad stretch (page 150)

Seated twist (page 115)

Sample Intermediate Workout, Focused on the Core

CARDIO

Begin with 20–40 minutes of cardio, such as walking briskly, jogging, or biking.

EXERCISES

Cat/cow (page 129)

Bridge (page 130)

Prone plank (page 132)

Supine plank (page 103)

Side plank (page 102)

Extended bicycle crunch (page 106)

Skater jumps (page 144)

Leg raises (page 135)

Superman (page 136)

Push-ups (page 141)

Medicine ball slams (page 110)

Skater jumps (second round)

Russian twists (page 111)

Lotus lift (page 88)

Medicine ball circles (page 143)

Stability ball pass (page 139)

Pigeon (page 87)

Butterfly (page 149)

Seated twist (page 115)

Quad stretch (page 150)

Sample Intermediate Workout, Focused on Strength

CARDIO

Begin with 20–40 minutes of cardio, or intersperse the cardio into your core/strength workout (for example, do jumping jacks or jog in place for 30 seconds between core exercises).

EXERCISES

Cat/cow (page 129)

Bridge (page 130)

Extended bicycle crunches (page 106)

Leg raises (page 135)

Side plank (page 102)

Push-ups (page 141)

Biceps curls (page 145)

Triceps extensions (page 146)

Around-the-world lunges (forward, side, backward) (page 148)

Squats (page 107)

Russian twists (page 111)

Superman (page 136)

Downward-facing dog (page 85)

Stability ball pass (page 139)

Supine ball twist (page 114)

Butterfly (page 149)

Seated twist (page 115)

Quad stretch (page 150)

Sample Advanced Workout

CARDIO

Begin with 30–45 minutes of cardio, or intersperse the cardio into your core/strength workout.

EXERCISES

Cat/cow (page 129)

Bridge (page 130)

Prone plank: 1 minute (page 132)

Supine plank: 1 minute (page 103)

Side plank: 30 seconds each side (page 102)

Push-ups on a balance trainer (page 141)

Bicycle crunches or extended bicycle crunches (page 134 or 106)

Squats on a balance trainer (page 107)

Superman (page 136)

Medicine ball slams (page 110)

Medicine ball pass (if workout buddy available) (page 113)

Russian twists (page 111)

Lotus lift (page 88)

Skater jumps with medicine ball (page 144)

Stability ball knee tuck (page 138)

Downward-facing dog (page 85)

Tree (page 84)

Supine ball twist (page 114)

Pigeon (page 87)

Butterfly (page 149)

Seated twist (page 115)

Quad stretch (page 150)

Sample Gym Workout (All Levels)

CARDIO

Warm up for 10 minutes by walking and/or jogging on a treadmill or using the elliptical.

EXERCISES

Leg raises (page 135)

Bicep curls (page 145)

Tricep extensions (page 146)

Forward lunges (page 147)

Side lunges (page 148)

Reverse lunges (page 147)

Squats (page 107)

Russian twists (page 111)

Prone plank (page 132)

Side plank (page 102)

Superman or swimmer (page 136 or 137)

Downward-facing dog (page 85)

Butterfly (page 149)

COREGASM 101 MENTAL MOTIVATION

I wrote earlier about how my favorite spin instructor tells us, "No challenge, no change!" This may seem corny, but it's motivational sayings like this that can keep many of us going when we'd prefer to give up. Here are some other mantras that have stuck with me:

- No challenge, no change.

- Success trains, failure complains.

- You can do this.

- I refuse to give up on myself.

- You can wake up sore or you can wake up sorry.

- You will never regret a workout.

- You don't get what you wish for; you get what you work for!

- Transformation lies on the other side of surrender.

- When you feel like quitting, think about why you started.

APPENDIX

Date: _____ Time: _____

Location: ☐ Gym ☐ Home ☐ Other: _____

C: Challenge yourself through cardio, reps, or resistance.

O: Order matters.

R: Relax and receive.

E: Engage your lower abdominals.

OVERALL SEQUENCE

Rate intensity from 1 (lowest) to 10 (highest)

1. Exercise Type: _____ Duration: _____ Intensity: _____ Response: A _____ O _____

2. Exercise Type: _____ Duration: _____ Intensity: _____ Response: A _____ O _____

3. Exercise Type: _____ Duration: _____ Intensity: _____ Response: A _____ O _____

4. Exercise Type: _____ Duration: _____ Intensity: _____ Response: A _____ O _____

Notes:

_____

_____

_____

_____

Cardio: □ Before Abs □ After Abs □ N/A

If Cardio Before Abs, how much time passed between cardio and abs? _____ min

Cardio length: _____ min

□ Running □ Elliptical □ Biking □ Stairmaster □ Other _____

Cardio intensity? (1 to 10; 1=not at all; 10=very): _____

A (1 to 10; 1=not at all; 10=very): _____ O: □ Yes □ No □ Close

If A, when: at _____ min

If O, when: at _____ min

EXERCISE 1: _____

Reps: _____ (_____ all at once? Or _____ sets of _____)

A (1 to 10; 1 = not at all; 10 = very): _____

O: □ Yes □ No □ Close

At what rep did A start? _____ At what rep O? _____

If weights: _____ lbs; □ light for you □ medium □ difficult

Notes:

_____

_____

_____

_____

EXERCISE 2: _____

Reps: _____ (_____ all at once? Or _____ sets of _____)

A (1 to 10; 1 = not at all; 10 = very): _____

O: □ Yes □ No □ Close

At what rep did A start? _____ At what rep O? _____

If weights: _____ lbs; □ light for you □ medium □ difficult

Notes:

_____

_____

_____

_____

COREGASM WORKOUT SURVEY

Are you a:

☐ Man ☐ Woman ☐ Transwoman (*male-to-female*) ☐ Transman (*female-to-male*)

What is your age? _____ years old

What made you decide to read *The Coregasm Workout?* (*Check all that apply.*)

☐ I was curious.

☐ I wanted to learn to experience exercise-induced arousal.

☐ I wanted to learn to experience exercise-induced orgasm.

☐ I've previously experienced exercise-induced arousal and wanted to learn more.

☐ I've previously experienced exercise-induced orgasms and wanted to learn more.

☐ Other (*Please describe*):

_____

_____

For those who've experienced exercise-induced orgasm:

If you have experienced orgasm during exercise, how old were you when it first occurred? _____ years old

What kind of exercising were you doing when it first occurred?

_____

Can you guess how many times you've experienced orgasm during exercise?
_____ times

Would you say that orgasms from exercise are:

☐ Easier for you, the stronger your core gets

☐ More difficult for you, the stronger your core gets

☐ There's no difference as far as you've noticed

For those who've tried the routines in this book:

If you have tried Coregasm Workout routines, about how many times have you done the exercises? _____ times

If you started experiencing arousal or orgasm after doing the Coregasm Workout routines, which exercises led to arousal?

_____

_____

_____

_____

Which exercises led to orgasms?

_____

_____

_____

_____

What aspects of the Coregasm Workout (either the C.O.R.E. Principles or the exercises themselves) worked for you?

_____

_____

_____

_____

What aspects of the Coregasm Workout (either the C.O.R.E. Principles or the exercises themselves) didn't work for you?

_____

_____

_____

_____

What other kinds of orgasms do you generally experience? (*Check all that apply.*)

☐ Orgasm from receiving oral sex

☐ Orgasm from penile-vaginal intercourse

☐ Orgasm from anal intercourse

☐ Orgasm during sleep or while dreaming

Is there anything else you would like to tell us?

_____

_____

_____

_____

THANK YOU!

You can mail the completed survey to:

Dr. Debby Herbenick

Department of Applied Health Science

School of Public Health, Room 116

1025 East 7th Street

Indiana University

Bloomington, IN 47405

USA

RESOURCES

To LEARN MORE about personal trainers and physical therapists and their certifying bodies, contact the following:

Aerobics and Fitness Association of America (AFAA)

15250 Ventura Boulevard, Suite 200

Sherman Oaks, CA 91403

www.afaa.com

American College of Sports Medicine (ACSM)

401 West Michigan Street

Indianapolis, IN 46202

www.acsm.org

(317) 637-9200

American Council on Exercise (ACE)

4851 Paramount Drive

San Diego, CA 92123

www.acefitness.org

(888) 825-3636

National Strength and Conditioning Association (NSCA)

1885 Bob Johnson Drive

Colorado Springs, CO 80906

www.nsca.com

(800) 815-6826

You can search for a sex therapist in your area by contacting the following:

American Association of Sexuality Educators, Counselors, and Therapists (AASECT)

1444 I Street, NW, Suite 700

Washington, DC 20005

www.aasect.org

(202) 449-1099

Society for Sex Therapy and Research

6311 W. Gross Point Road

Niles, IL 60714

www.sstarnet.org

(847) 647-8832

NOTES

Introduction

many women masturbated: A. Kinsey, W. Pomeroy, C. Martin, and P. Gebhard, *Sexual Behavior in the Human Female* (Philadelphia: W.B. Saunders, 1953), 176-190.

different ways to experience orgasm: B.R. Komisaruk and B. Whipple, "Non-Genital Orgasms," *Sexual and Relationship Therapy* 26, no. 4 (2011): 356–372.

Chapter 1: The Curious Case of the Coregasm

the term coregasm: "More Than Squat," April 18, 2007, accessed August 1, 2014, http://pagesix.com/2007/04/18/more-than-squat.

"A Good Reason to Work Your Core," April 18, 2007, accessed August 1, 2014, http://pastaqueen.com/blog/2007/04/a-good-reason-to-work-your-core.

"The Simple Leg Exercise That Could Replace Your Vibrator," April 18, 2007, accessed August 1, 2014, www.celebitchy.com/3644/the_simple_leg_exercise_that_could_replace _your_vibrator.

sexual variety increases potential for orgasm: D. Herbenick, M. Reece, V. Schick, S.A. Sanders, B. Dodge, &, J.D Fortenberry, "An Event-Level Analysis of the Sexual Characteristics and Composition Among Adults Ages 18 to 59: Results from a National Probability Sample in the United States," *Journal of Sexual Medicine* 7, suppl 5 (2010): 346–361, accessed November 18, 2014, doi: 10.1111/j.1743-6109.2010.02020.x.

reassure parents: See for example, "Caring For Your School-Aged Child: Ages 5 to 12," American Academy of Pediatrics, accessed November 18, 2014, www.healthychildren. org/English/ages-stages/gradeschool/puberty/Pages/Masturbation.aspx; and "Talking with Your Young Child about Sex," American Academy of Pediatrics, accessed November 18, 2014, http://patiented.aap.org/content2.aspx?aid=5063.

and some men: Although most men experience orgasm easily during sex with a partner, some men experience what is called "delayed ejaculation, or DE" or "inhibited ejaculation, or IE," which is when it either takes a very long time for them to ejaculate (as with DE) or else they try and are unable to ejaculate (as with IE). Sex therapists can help with both of these issues; to find a sex therapist in your area, see the Resources section in the Appendix.

trying to increase strength: D.G. Behm, E.J. Drinkwater, J.M. Willardson, and P.M. Cowley, "Canadian Society for Exercise Physiology Position Stand: The Use of Instability to Train the Core in Athletic and Nonathletic Conditioning," *Applied Physiology, Nutrition, and Metabolism* 35 (2010): 109–112.

Chapter 3: C.O.R.E. Principle #1

great spectacle at the circus: from Daniel P. Mannix, *Those About to Die* (New York: Random House, 1974), 26–27.

activation of the SNS can enhance women's sexual arousal: Meston, C.M. (2000). Sympathetic nervous system activity and female sexual arousal. *American Journal of Cardiology*, 86 (suppl): 30F–34F.

exercise at least twice a week: U.S. Department of Health and Human Services, Office of Disease Prevention and Health Promotion, 2008 Physical Activity Guidelines for Americans Summary, accessed October 25, 2014, www.health.gov/paguidelines/guidelines/summary.aspx.

giving your muscles time to recover: G. Kolata, "WELL; Personal Best: Workouts Have Their Limits, Recognized or Not," *The New York Times,* January 7, 2012, accessed October 25, 2014, http://query.nytimes.com/gst/fullpage.html?res=9D05E5D71F31F934 A25752C0A9649D8B63.

Chapter 4: C.O.R.E. Principle #2

"gentle wake-ups" for your spine: V. Akuthota, A. Ferreiro, T. Moore, and M. Fredericson, Core stability exercise principles, *Current Sports Medicine Reports* 7, no. 1 (2008): 39–44.

Chapter 5: C.O.R.E. Principle #3

male smokers with erectile dysfunction: E. Oksuz and S. Malhan, Prevalence and Risk Factors for Female Sexual Dysfunction in Turkish Women," *The Journal of Urology* 175 (2006): 654–658. See also G. Pourmand, M.R. Alidaee, S. Rasuli, A. Maleki, and A. Mehrsai, "Do Cigarette Smokers with Erectile Dysfunction Benefit From Stopping? A Prospective Study," *BJU International,* 94 (2004): 1310–1313. See also C.B. Harte and C.M. Meston, "The Inhibitory Effects of Nicotine on Physiological Sexual Arousal in Nonsmoking Women: Results from a Randomized, Double-Blind, Placebo-Controlled, Cross-Over Trial," *Journal of Sexual Medicine* 5 (2008): 1184–1197.

like mindfulness, tantra, and yoga: L. Brotto, L. Mehak, and C. Kit, "Yoga and Sexual Functioning: A Review," *Journal of Sex & Marital Therapy,* 35 (2009): 378–390.

yoga benefits our physical health: See for example: Hadi, N., & Hadi, N. (2007). Effects of hatha yoga on well-being in healthy adults in Shiraz, Islamic Republic of Iran. *Eastern Mediterranean Health Journal,* 13, 829–837; Krishnamurthy, M. N., & Telles, S. (2007). Assessing depression following two ancient Indian interventions: Effects of yoga and ayurveda on older adults in a residential home. *Journal of Gerontological Nursing,* 33, 17–23; McCaffrey, R., Ruknui, P., Hatthakit, U., & Kasetsomboon, P. (2005). The effects of yoga on hypertensive persons in Thailand. *Holistic Nursing Practice,* 19, 173–180; Prakash, S., Meshram, S., & Ramtekkar, U. (2007). Athletes, yogis and individuals with sedentary lifestyles; Do their lung functions differ? *Indian Journal of Physiology and Pharmacology,* 51, 76–80; Shapiro, D., Cook, I. A., Davydov, D. M., Ottaviani, C., Leuchter, A. F., & Abrams, M. (2007). Yoga as a complementary treatment of depression: Effects of traits and moods on treatment outcome. *Evidence Based Complementary and Alternative Medicine,* 4, 493–502.; Smith, C., Hancock, H., Blake-Mortimer, J., & Eckert, K. (2007). A randomized comparative trial of yoga and relaxation to reduce stress and anxiety. *Complementary Therapies in Medicine,* 15, 77–83; Smith, K. B., & Pukall, C. F. (2009). An evidence-based review of yoga as a complementary intervention for patients with cancer. *Psychooncology,* 18, 465–475.

yoga and premature ejaculation and ejaculatory control in men: Dhikav, V., Karmarkar, G., Gupta, M., & Anand, K. S. (2007). Yoga in premature ejaculation: A comparative trial with fluoxetine. *Journal of Sexual Medicine, 4,* 1726–1732.

yoga and sexual desire, lubrication, and arousal in women: V. Dhikav, G. Karmarkar, R. Gupta, M. Verma, R. Gupta, S. Gupta, and K.S.Anand, "Yoga in Female Sexual Functions," *Journal of Sexual Medicine* 7 (2010): 964–970.

among Korean women with metabolic syndrome: H.N. Kim, J. Ryu, K.S. Kim, and S.W. Song, "Effects of Yoga on Sexual Function in Women with Metabolic Syndrome: a Randomized Controlled Trial, *Journal of Sexual Medicine* 10 (2013): 2741–2751.

prefrontal cortex and meditative states and female orgasm: A. Chiesa and A. Serretti, "A Systematic Review of Neurobiological and Clinical Features of Mindfulness Meditations., *Psychological Medicine* 40, no. 8 (2010): 1239–1252.

orgasm through thought alone: For a discussion of this research, see K. Sukel, "Sex on the Brain: Orgasms Unlock Altered Consciousness," *New Scientist*, May 11, 2011, accessed October 25, 2014, www.newscientist.com/article/mg21028124.600-sex-on-the-brain-orgasms-unlock-altered-consciousness.html#.VE5lMou_ioY.

yoga, attention, and breathing: See for example: Gupta, N., Khera, S., Vempati, R. P., Sharma, R., & Bijlani, R. L. (2006). Effect of yoga based lifestyle intervention on state and trait anxiety. Indian Journal of Physiology and Pharmacology, 50, 41–47; Telles, S., Raghuraj, P., Arankalle, D., & Naveen, K. V. (2008). Immediate effect of high-frequency yoga breathing on attention. Indian Journal of Medical Sciences, 62, 20–22.

yoga: less stressed or anxious: McAffrey, R., Ruknui, P., Hatthakit, U., and Kasetsomboon, P. (2005). The effects of yoga on hypertensive persons in Thailand. Holistic Nursing Practice, 19(4), 173-180. Michalsen, A., Grossman, P., Acil, A., Langhorst, J., Ludtke, R., Esch, T., Stefano, G. B., & Dobos, G. J. (2005). Rapid stress reduction and anxiolysis among distressed women as a consequence of a three-month intensive yoga program. *Medical Science Monitor:* International Medical Journal of Experimental and Clinical Research, 11, CR555–561; Smith, C., Hancock, H., Blake-Mortimer, J., & Eckert, K. (2007). A randomized comparative trial of yoga and relaxation to reduce stress and anxiety. *Complementary Therapies in Medicine*, 15, 77–83.

relaxed conditions: See Krishnamurthy MN, Telles S. Assessing depression following two ancient Indian interventions: Effects of yoga and ayurveda on older adults in a residential home. J Gerontol Nurs 2007;33:17–23; See also McAffrey, R., Ruknui, P., Hatthakit, U., and Kasetsomboon, P. (2005). The effects of yoga on hypertensive persons in Thailand. *Holistic Nursing Practice,* 19(4), 173-180.

yoga: easier arousal, more pleasurable sex: Metz, M.E. and McCarthy, B.W. (2007). The "Good Enough Sex Model" for couple sexual satisfaction. Sexual and relationship therapy, 22(3), 351–362.

yoga, positive feelings, and life satisfaction: Impett, E. A., Daubenmier, J. J., & Hirschman, A. L. (2006). Minding the body: Yoga, embodiment and well-being. *Sexuality Research & Social Policy,* 3, 39–48.

mindfulness training can help us to reduce stress: Scientific research on mindful meditation practices has found that such practices can result in less stress, lower blood pressure, and enhancement of areas of the brain related to attention. See A. Chiesa and A. Serretti, "A Systematic Review of Neurobiological and Clinical Features of Mindfulness Meditations," *Psychological Medicine* 40, no. 8 (2010): 1239–1252.

psychologist Lori Brotto found: L. Brotto, R. Basson, and M. Luria, "A Mindfulness-Based Group Psychoeducational Intervention Targeting Sexual Arousal Disorder in Women," *Journal of Sexual Medicine* 5, no. 7 (2008): 1646–1659.

women prone to "cognitive distractions" during sex: Barlow, D. H. (1986). Causes of sexual dysfunction: The role of anxiety and cognitive interference. *Journal of Consulting and Clinical Psychology,* 54, 140–148.

Dove, N. L., & Wiederman, M.W. (2000). Cognitive distraction and women's sexual functioning. *Journal of Sex and Marital Therapy,* 26, 67–78.

Chapter 6: C.O.R.E. Principle #4

G-spot and precise scientific understanding: For a more in-depth discussion of the G-Spot than we can fit here, check out my earlier book, *Sex Made Easy: Your Awkward Questions Answered for Better, Smarter, Amazing Sex* (Philadelphia: Running Press,

2012). See also A.K. Ladas, B. Whipple, and J. Perry, *The G Spot: And Other Discoveries in Human Sexuality* (New York: Henry Holt and Company, 1982).

twenty-nine pairs of muscles/sort of box: V. Akuthota, A. Ferreiro, T. Moore, and M. Fredericson, "Core Stability Exercise Principles," *Current Sports Medicine Reports* 7, no. 1 (2008): 39–44.

adjust or avoid certain sex positions: N.S. Sidorkewicz and S.M. McGill, "Male Spine Motion During Coitus: Implications for the Low Back Pain Patient," *Spine* 39, no. 20 (2014): 1633–1639.

Speaking, laughing, coughing: A. DeTroyer, M. Estenne, V. Ninane, D. Van Gansbeke, and M. Gorini. "Transversus Abdominis Muscle Function in Humans," *Journal of Applied Physiology* 68 no. 3 (1990): 1010–1016.

Pilates exercises engage TrA: I. Endleman and D.J. Critchley, "Transversus Abdominis and Obliques Internus Activity During Pilates Exercises: Measurement with Ultrasound Scanning," *Archives of Physical Medicine and Rehabilitation* 89 (2008): 2205–2212.

core works together as a unit: T. Nesser, K.C. Huxel, J.L. Tincher, and T. Okada, "The Relationship Between Core Stability and Performance in Division 1 Football Players," *The Journal of Strength & Conditioning Research* 22, no. 6 (2008): 1750–1754.

no single exercise engages every core muscle: S.M. McGill, *Ultimate Back Fitness and Performance,* 4th ed. (Waterloo, Ontario: Backfit Pro, Inc., 2009).

no single core exercise routine will suit everyone: C.T. Axler and S.M. McGill, "Low Back Loads over a Variety of Abdominal Exercises: Searching for the Safest Abdominal Challenge," *Medicine and Science in Sports and Exercise* 29, no. 6 (1997): 804–811.

Experts in spine health: M.A. Adams, P. Dolan, and W.C. Hutton, "Diurnal Variations in the Stresses on the Lumbar Spine," *Spine* 12, no. 2 (1987): 130–137.

planks engage the lower abdominal muscles: D.G. Behm, A.M. Leonard, W.B. Young, W.A. Bonsey, and S.N. MacKinnon, "Trunk Muscle Electromyographic Activity with Unstable and Unilateral Exercises," *Journal of Strength and Conditioning Research* 19, no. 1 (2005): 193–201.

Twists involve trunk rotation and engage core: J.M. Martuscello, J.L. Nuzzo, C.D. Ashley, B.I. Campbell, J.J. Orrioloa, and J.M. Mayer, "Systematic Review of Core Muscle Activity During Physical Fitness Exercises," *Journal of Strength and Conditioning Research* 27, no. 6 (2013): 1684–1698.

diaphragmatic breathing techniques and pelvic floor activation: R. Sapsford, "Explanation of Medical Terminology," *Neurourology and Urodynamics* 19, no. 5 (2000): 633. See also, P.B. O'Sullivan, D.J. Beales, J.A. Beetham, et al., "Altered Motor Control Strategies in Subjects with Sacroiliac Joint Pain During the Active Straight-Leg-Raise Test," *Spine* 27 (2002): E1–E8. See also V. Akuthota, A. Ferreiro, T. Moore, and M. Fredericson, "Core Stability Exercise Principles," *Current Sports Medicine Reports* 7, no. 1 (2008): 39–44.

. . . other difficulties: J.S. Petrofsky, M. Cuneo, R. Dial, and A. Morris, "Muscle Activity during Yoga Breathing Exercise Compared to Abdominal Crunches," *The Journal of Applied Research* 5, no. 3 (2005): 501–507.

Pilates and pelvic floor muscle training (PFMT): P.J. Culligan, J. Scherer, K. Dyer, J.L. Priestley, G. Guingon-White, D. Delvecchio, and M. Vangeli, "A Randomized Clinical Trial Comparing Pelvic Floor Muscle Training to a Pilates Exercise Program for Improved Pelvic Muscle Strength," *International Urogynecology Journal* 21 (2010): 401–408.

2008 New Zealand study: N. Dean, D. Wilson, P. Herbison, C. Glazener, T. Aung, and, C. Macarthur, "Sexual Function, Delivery Mode History, Pelvic Floor Muscle Exercises, and Incontinence: A Cross-Sectional Study Six Years Post-Partum," *New Zealand Journal of Obstetrics and Gynaecology* 48 (2008): 302–311.

improve sexual desire and likelihood of orgasm: P.A. Roughan and L. Knust, "Do Pelvic Floor Exercises Really Improve Orgasmic Potential?," *Journal of Sex & Marital Therapy* 7 (1981): 223–229. See also M.R. Messé and J.H. Greer, "Voluntary Vaginal Musculature Contractions as an Enhancer of Sexual Arousal," *Archives of Sexual Behavior* 14, (1985): 13–28.

strain during childbirth: "The Controversy Over Kegels: Are Women Doing Them Correctly?," *The Alexander Foundation for Women's Health*, June 2004, accessed August 20, 2014, www.afwh.org/articles/paid/controversyoverkegels.htm. Dr. Whipple is a well-known nurse and sexuality researcher who has spent her career furthering our understanding of female sexuality; Ms. Rosenbaum is a well-regarded physical therapist and sex therapist.

don't "practice" stopping your urine: Mayo Clinic Staff, "Kegel Exercises: A How-to Guide for Women," Mayo Clinic, September 25, 2012, accessed November 18, 2014, www. mayoclinic.org/healthy-living/womens-health/in-depth/kegel-exercises/art-20045283.

most demanding exercise is pelvic tilting: Monfort-Panego, M., Vera-Garcia, F.J., Sanchez-Zuriaga, D., and Sarti-Martinez, M.A. Electromyographic studies in abdominal exercises: a literature synthesis. *Journal of Manipulative and Physiological Therapeutics*, 32(3), 232-244.

Chapter 7: The Coregasm Workout Exercises and Routines

work out more often . . . higher grades: X.S. Keating, D. Castelli, and S.F. Ayers, "Association of Weekly Strength Exercise Frequency and Academic Performance Among Students at a Large University in the United States," *Journal of Strength and Conditioning Research* 27, no. 3, (2013): 1988–1993.

improve mood and lower depression: R. Stanton and P. Reaburn, "Exercise and the Treatment of Depression: A Review of the Exercise Program Variables," *Journal of Science and Medicine in Sport* 17, no. 2 (2014): 177–182.

higher bone density: W. Kemmler and S. von Stengel, "Dose-Response Effect of Exercise Frequency on Bone Mineral Density in Post-Menopausal, Osteopenic Women," *Scandinavian Journal of Medicine & Science in Sports* 24, no. 3 (2014): 526–534.

recognized certifying bodies: D. Bradley, "Most Recognized Personal Training Certifications," *Livestrong.com,* last modified December 20, 2010, accessed November 18, 2014,www.livestrong.com/article/339261-most-recognized-personal-training-certifications.

ACKNOWLEDGMENTS

I AM FORTUNATE TO have had a stellar team to work with in creating *The Coregasm Workout.* *I* am forever thankful to my literary agent, Kari Stuart at ICM, for believing that exercise-induced orgasms are not only real but experiences that many people have questions about and, of course, for shepherding this book to a point where it, too, could become real and help people. I am grateful to Laura Mazer, my editor at Seal Press, who was intrigued by the concept and has believed in the possibilities of sex and exercise to influence one another. Thank you, Laura, for your unwavering support. Merrik Bush-Pirkle and Kirsten Janene-Nelson were so helpful with their close edits and thoughtful suggestions. I feel lucky to have worked with them both. Seal has so many terrific people: Tabitha Lahr and Jane Musser produced a beautiful book that I'm proud to hold in my hands and share with the world. And I am also appreciative of Eva Zimmerman, my publicist, who took the time to understand what *The Coregasm Workout* is about and helps me share that vision with others. The images of the core muscles are thanks to Tom Weinzerl in the Office of Visual Media at Indiana University.

At IU's School of Public Health, anything is possible. Michael Reece and David Koceja were among the first researchers I asked for advice about studying EIO/EIA – namely, whether they knew people who studied exercise and muscle movements and who might be able to pair their expertise with mine. They saw value in this research and encouraged my early work, and I owe many thanks to each of them. I am also indebted to my friend Scott Butler, a professor at Georgia College and State University, who introduced me to his colleague, Chris Black (now at the University of Oklahoma), who has further helped me put together the pieces of the EIO/EIA puzzle. Chris, thank you for not even blinking the first time I shared with you what I hoped to study (and thanks, too, for your time, support, and sharing of your expertise).

Dan Savage helped me distribute my first exercise-induced orgasm and arousal (EIO/EIA) study, which allowed me to quickly find hundreds of people who were willing to share their stories. Dan is a powerful voice and a great person and if you don't yet listen to his Savage Love podcasts or read his column, you're missing out. Shortly after I finished my first EIO/EIA survey, I shared the results with one of my closest colleagues and mentors at IU, Dennis Fortenberry. I asked if he'd join me on this interesting journey to understand EIO/EIA, and he (thankfully) agreed. Everyone needs someone in their lives to listen to their ideas and support them, and Dennis has often been that person for me. Similarly, Georgia Frey (a kinesiology professor at IU) has been one of my strongest allies and co-investigators in this research. During the summer of 2013, she let me take over her lab space and move exercise equipment into it and paired me with two smart and easy-to-talk-with graduate students (who also happened to work as personal trainers), Freddie Holmgren and Susie Owen, who were my co-interviewers in one of our EIO/EIA studies. I can't say enough positive things about the intelligence, thoughtfulness, and compassion these women brought to our interviews. I am also thankful to Brady Singleton and Antonio Williams, who have been terrific sounding boards for ideas. Their knowledge of exercise science has been so helpful. Additionally, I am grateful to Meredith Davis, Roshni Dhoot, and Elizabeth Day for their assistance on one of our EIO/EIA studies. I would like to thank Beverly Whipple for encouraging me to explore and better understand the diverse ways in which human beings experience orgasm.

Throughout the process of studying "coregasm" and writing this book, I immersed myself in research conducted and published by many well-respected scientists who study exercise and the core muscles. In particular, I read a great deal of work by Drs. Venu Akuthota, Stuart McGill, Natalie Sidorkewicz , Tamara Moore, Jason Martuscello, Garry Allison, Brendan Lay, and many more. Anything I got right about muscles and exercise is because of their wisdom and research; any shortcomings are my own.

The women of Bloomington, Indiana came together to help make this book a reality. Bianca, Diana, Freddie, Holly, Janay, Jill, and Valerie graciously agreed to be fitness models for *The Coregasm Workout*. These are real women who exercise in their everyday lives. Chelsea Sanders of Blueline Media in Bloomington, Indiana photographed us. Our hair was by Chelsea Langley and makeup was by Julie McLenachen at Royale Hair

Parlor in Bloomington, Indiana (many thanks to salon owner Bridgett DiVohl for her support).

I owe a thousand thanks to Jill Rensink. As my personal trainer (and someone who is smart and thoughtful about the human body and exercise), Jill has patiently listened to me ponder the mysteries of coregasm, and our research about this interesting phenomenon. Jill also consulted on the book by reviewing the exercises in The Coregasm Workout, advising me on how to word some of the directions and cues, and overseeing our form during the photo shoot. Jill is the real deal: a lifetime athlete, she's competed in gymnastics, track and field, cross country, and road racing. In college at Iowa State University, she competed as an NCAA Division I athlete in track and field and graduated with a degree in sports marketing. Jill has been an ACE (American Council on Exercise) Certified Personal Trainer since 2006 and also holds certifications in TRX and BOSU and is generally just super smart, encouraging, and awesome. I'm so grateful she was willing to work on this project with me.

I owe an enormous debt of gratitude to the thousands of women and men who have generously shared of themselves by participating in our research studies. Without them, none of this would be possible. Thank you.

My mom is the one who first got me (as a child) interested in exercise. She took my sister and I to her aerobics classes and tennis matches. She and our dad taught us to swim as soon as we could walk and to play tennis, baseball (our best games were in Maine), ride bikes, and to dance. We had an active, fun childhood and I learned to love exercise at an early age thanks to them (and thanks to Olivia Newton-John's smash hit "Let's Get Physical" that was popular when I was a kid.)

I'd like to thank friends and colleagues like Michael, Brian, Vanessa, Jenny, Catherine, Shawn, Pat and all of our graduate students at the Center for Sexual Health Promotion and The Kinsey Institute who have been supportive of this research. And I would be lost without the love and friendship of Brad, Brian, Catherine, Erica, Erin, James, Jarrett, Jenny, Jezebel, Lydia, Mallory, Maureen, and Sally, all of my fun book club friends, and Rick. Thank you.

ABOUT THE AUTHOR

Dr. DEBBY HERBENICK is an internationally known sex researcher, educator, columnist, and author. She is an associate professor at Indiana University's School of Public Health and a research fellow and sexual health educator for the Kinsey Institute

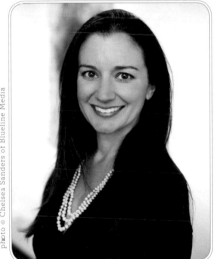

photo © Chelsea Sanders of Blueline Media

for Research in Sex, Gender, and Reproduction. She holds a PhD in Health Behavior from Indiana University, a master's degree in Public Health from Indiana University, and a bachelor's degree in Psychology from the University of Maryland. She is also certified as a sexuality educator by the American Association of Sexuality Educators, Counselors, and Therapists. Dr. Herbenick has published more than ninety scientific articles about sexual health, behavior, sexual arousal, and orgasm, and has written five books about sex and love. Originally from Miami, Florida, she currently lives and works in Bloomington, Indiana.

INDEX

SELECTED TITLES FROM SEAL PRESS

Yogalosophy: 28 Days to the Ultimate Mind-Body Makeover, by Mandy Ingber. $18.00, 978-1-58005-445-4. Celebrity yoga instructor Mandy Ingber offers a realistic, flexible, daily plan that will help readers transform their minds, their bodies, and their lives.

The 3-Day Reset: Restore Your Cravings For Healthy Foods in Three Easy, Empowering Days, by Pooja Mottl. $22.00, 978-1-58005-527-7. These 10 simple resets target and revamp your eating habits in practical, three-day increments.

Book Lovers: Sexy Stories from Under the Covers, edited by Shawna Kenney. $15.00, 978-1-58005-529-1. Both sexy and smart, this anthology of intelligent erotica is written by and for literature lovers.

What You Can When You Can: 50 Ways to Reach Your Healthy Living Goals, by Carla Birnberg and Roni Noone. $10.00, 978-1-58005-573-4. This companion book to the #wycwyc movement teaches you to harness the power of small steps to achieve your health and fitness goals.

Prude: Lessons I Learned When My Fiancé Filmed Porn, by Emily Southwood. $16.00, 978-1-58005-498-0. This humorous memoir reveals the author's bizarre journey to conquer her discomfort around porn—and how she ends up finding herself and ultimately fixing her relationship for good along the way.

Sexual Intimacy for Women: A Guide for Same-Sex Couples, by Glenda Corwin, PhD $16.95, 978-1-58005-303-7. In this prescriptive and poignant book, Glenda Corwin, PhD, helps female couples overcome obstacles to sexual intimacy through her examination of the emotional, physical, and psychological aspects of same-sex relationships.

Find Seal Press Online
www.sealpress.com
www.facebook.com/sealpress
Twitter: @SealPress